CyberGenetics

Online genetic testing services are increasingly being offered to consumers who are becoming exposed to, and knowledgeable about, new kinds of genetic technologies, as the launch of a 23andMe genetic testing product in the United Kingdom testifies. Genetic research breakthroughs, cheek-swabbing forensic pathologists, and celebrities discovering their ancestral roots are littered throughout the North American, European and Australasian media landscapes. Genetic testing is now capturing the attention, and imagination, of hundreds of thousands of people who can not only buy genetic tests online, but can also go online to find relatives, share their results with strangers, sign up for personal DNA-based musical scores, and take part in research. This book critically examines this market of direct-to-consumer (DTC) genetic testing from a social science perspective, asking: 'What happens when genetics goes online?'

With a focus on genetic testing for disease, the book is about the new social arrangements which emerge when a traditionally clinical practice (genetic testing) is taken into new spaces (the internet). It examines the intersections of new genetics and new media by drawing from three different fields: internet studies, the sociology of health, and science and technology studies.

While there has been a surge of research activity concerning DTC genetic testing, particularly in sociology, ethics and law, this is the first scholarly monograph on the topic, and the first book which brings together the social study of genetics and the social study of digital technologies. This book thus not only offers a new overview of this field, but also offers a unique contribution by attending to the digital, and by drawing upon empirical examples from our own research of DTC genetic testing websites (using online methods) and in-depth interviews in the UK with people using healthcare services.

Anna Harris completed a medical degree at the University of Tasmania, and a Masters and PhD in medical anthropology at the University of Melbourne. She has been a post-doctoral researcher at the Universities of Maastricht and Exeter. She has published in clinical and social science journals, and has her own blog.

Susan Kelly is Associate Professor of medical sociology at the University of Exeter, and Senior Research Fellow in Egenis (Exeter Centre for the Study of the Life Sciences). She earned a PhD in sociology at the University of California, San Francisco, followed by a post-doctoral position in the Stanford Center for Biomedical Ethics.

Sally Wyatt is Programme Leader of the e-Humanities Group at the Royal Netherlands Academy of Arts and Sciences, and Professor of digital cultures in development at Maastricht University. She is the founding co-editor (with Andrew Webster) of the Health, Technology and Society series published by Palgrave Macmillan.

Genetics and Society

Series editors: Ruth Chadwick, former Director of Cesagene, Cardiff University; John Dupré, Director of Egenis, University of Exeter and University of Edinburgh; David Wield, Director of Innogen, Edinburgh University; and Steve Yearley, former Director of the Genomics Forum, Edinburgh University.

The books in this series, all based on original research, explore the social, economic and ethical consequences of the new genetic sciences. The series is based in Cesagene, one of the centres forming the ESRC's Genomics Network (EGN), the largest UK investment in social science research on the implications of these innovations. With a mix of research monographs, edited collections, textbooks and a major new handbook, the series is a valuable contribution to the social analysis of developing and emergent biotechnologies.

Series titles include:

New Genetics, New Social Formations
Peter Glasner, Paul Atkinson and Helen Greenslade

New Genetics, New Identities
Paul Atkinson, Peter Glasner and Helen Greenslade

The GM Debate
Risk, politics and public engagement
Tom Horlick-Jones, John Walls, Gene Rowe, Nick Pidgeon, Wouter Poortinga, Graham Murdock and Tim O'Riordan

Growth Cultures
Life sciences and economic development
Philip Cooke

Human Cloning in the Media
Joan Haran, Jenny Kitzinger, Maureen McNeil and Kate O'Riordan

Local Cells, Global Science
Embryonic stem cell research in India
Aditya Bharadwaj and Peter Glasner

Handbook of Genetics and Society
Paul Atkinson, Peter Glasner and Margaret Lock

The Human Genome
Chamundeeswari Kuppuswamy

The merger of information technology and genetics into 'cybergenetics' is an important development in health science. This book offers crucial critical insights into revamped versions of genetic determinism, the role of online platforms and companies in medical research, and questions of trust with regards to the digital technologies that increasingly organize our healthcare. Harris, Kelly and Wyatt provide a much needed guide to the cybergenetics future.

José van Dijck, Professor of Media Studies, University of Amsterdam

Genetics has long remained an obscure field, carefully hidden from public consciousness. Now, in contrast, it is has become both mainstream and big business. Typically, genetic results for humans are highly personal and intensively political at the same time. Through its mixed and playful methodology and its broad theoretical framing, *CyberGenetics* demonstrates how the public view of genetic testing and personal genomics – as seen through social media and the Internet – revolves around several explosive axes: privacy vs. exposure, fear vs. hope, participation vs. exploitation. This book has much to offer for those interested in the exploration of identity, self and belonging through the examination of genetic avenues and informed debates about science and politics.

Gísli Pálsson, Professor Semi-Emeritus,
Department of Anthropology, University of Iceland

This book is a powerful antidote to simplistic portrayals of online genetics as either empowering or harming test-takers. Using novel and innovative methodologies to explore how users and health professionals make sense of online genetics, it provides fascinating and also troubling insights into the meaning of online genetics at the personal, social, and political levels.

Barbara Prainsack, Professor of Sociology,
Department of Social Science, Health & Medicine, King's College London

In *CyberGenetics*, Anna Harris, Susan Kelly and Sally Wyatt have successfully combined close reading of an impressive body of work from science and technology studies, internet studies, and the sociology of health and illness, with a deep knowledge of trends and developments in direct-to-consumer genetic testing. They offer us a critical and rigorous account of how genetic and digital worlds are remaking each other and, along the way, experiment with writing in alternative voices, from autobiologies, future scenarios, to poetry. The result is an enjoyable, thoughtful, and imaginative book, which offers an indispensable guide to non-experts, students, and researchers wishing to make sense of what happens when genetics goes online.

Richard Tutton, Senior Lecturer,
Department of Sociology, Lancaster University

CyberGenetics

Health genetics and new media

Anna Harris, Susan Kelly and Sally Wyatt

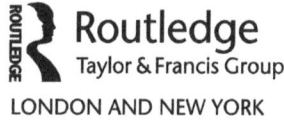

Routledge
Taylor & Francis Group

LONDON AND NEW YORK

First published 2016 by Routledge

2 Park Square, Milton Park, Abingdon, Oxfordshire OX14 4RN
711 Third Avenue, New York, NY 10017

Routledge is an imprint of the Taylor & Francis Group, an informa business

First issued in paperback 2018

British Library Cataloguing-in-Publication Data
A catalogue record for this book is available from the British Library

Library of Congress Cataloging-in-Publication Data
Names: Harris, Anna (Medical anthropologist) | Kelly, Susan (Susan Elizabeth)
| Wyatt, Sally, 1959–
Title: Cybergenetics : health genetics and new media / by Anna Harris, Susan
Kelly, Sally Wyatt.
Other titles: Cyber genetics
Description: Abingdon, Oxon ; New York, NY : Routledge, 2016.
Identifiers: LCCN 2015040927| ISBN 9781138946514 (hardback) | ISBN
9781315670799 (ebook)
Subjects: LCSH: Human chromosome abnormalities—Diagnosis—Computer
network resources. | Genetic screening—Computer network resources. | Genetic
screening—Social aspects. | Internet.
Classification: LCC RB155.65 .K45 2016 | DDC 362.196/04207—dc23
LC record available at http://lccn.loc.gov/2015040927

ISBN: 978-1-138-94651-4 (hbk)
ISBN: 978-1-138-35193-6 (pbk)

Typeset in Times New Roman
by FiSH Books Ltd, Enfield

For Thomas, Stephen and Hans

Contents

Acknowledgements

Much academic work is solitary, but we have been lucky enough to work together in the preparation of this book, and to benefit from the knowledge, skills and experience of each other. It has been an enormous pleasure to do so. We have also benefitted from the support and insights of many others.

Let's start with the money, as it is the case that without financial support we could not have started much less finished this project. This research was supported by the Bilateral Agreement Scheme between the Economic and Social Research Council (grant number ES/H0250330/1 (Kelly)/RES-000-22-3864), and the Netherlands Organisation for Scientific Research (grant number 463-09-033). The title that appeared on the project application was 'Selling Genetic Tests Online: User Perspectives on Direct to Consumer Psychiatric Genetic Tests'. We did indeed address those issues, but the project went in other very interesting directions, and we are grateful for the freedom the funding gave us to pursue those. The project formally lasted for two years, from December 2010 to November 2012.

We received additional financial support from both the Research Stimulation Fund of the Faculty of Arts and Social Sciences at Maastricht University, and from Universiteits Fonds Limburg/SWOL. This enabled us to host a group of international scholars working on related themes for a workshop we organised in September 2012 in Maastricht, called 'Genetics Goes Online'. We also received funding for open access publication from the NWO, and the University of Exeter.

We collectively received a writing fellowship from the Brocher Foundation in Hermance, Switzerland, that gave us the opportunity to be together for a whole month in the spring of 2015. We seized the chance to work together closely in a beautiful environment, in order to make substantial progress on this book. We are extremely grateful to the Scientific Committee of the Foundation for their belief in our project, and to the staff and our fellow fellows for helping to make our stay both enjoyable and productive. While in Switzerland, we benefitted from the hospitality and inspiration provided by Marc Audétat, and his colleagues at Université de Lausanne.

This brings us to the many people who have helped us in myriad ways during the years we have worked on this project. Many people have commented upon drafts of texts, asked questions during presentations, proffered advice and suggestions, and given practical support. We are grateful to them all for their personal and unique contributions, but here can only proffer an alphabetical list: Samantha Adams (co-author on TCS paper; see below), Roland Bal, Alyson Claffey, Julian Cockbain, Anja de Haas, John Dupré, Christopher Elphick, Jan Hodgson, Ine van Hoyweghen, Arthur Frank, Jan Frich, Sandra Lee, Sabina Leonelli, Wilma Lieben, Andreas Mitzschke, Michael Morrison, Gísli Pálsson, Bart van Oost, Barbara Prainsack, Evelyn Ruppert, Tamar Sharon, Heather Skirton, Sigrid Sterckx, and Ties van der Werff. Many anonymous reviewers have also generously shared their insights without expectation of personal recognition, but we appreciate their efforts. On a more collective level, we are grateful to our colleagues in MUSTS (Maastricht University STS), and Egenis (now the Exeter Centre for the Study of Life Sciences), and the Genomics Network (ESRC funded), for providing such collegial working environments. We would also like to thank colleagues throughout the ESRC Genomics Network for their inspiring and helpful work, and for reviewing versions of the proposal for this book. Kelly would like to thank members of the sociology of diagnosis network, and the Health, Technology and Society (HTS) research group at Exeter.

Anonymous interview participants generously provided their time and thoughts, and we thank them for sharing those with us. We would also like to thank Andy Gibson of the PenCLARC (Penninsula Collaboration for Leadership in Applied Health Research and Care), and the PenPIG (Penninsula Patient Involvement Group) at the University of Exeter, and the members of the patient involvement group he organised to provide input into our interviews.

We are grateful to our colleague in Maastricht, Caoilinn Hughes, for writing the poem 'Predictive Measures' for the Conclusion. We are also grateful to her for permission to use 'Apple Falls from the Tree', originally published in *New Poetries VI: An Anthology of Verse*, published by Carcanet Press (Manchester) in 2015. More of Caoilinn's poetry, often inspired by past, and contemporary scientific developments, can be found in *Gathering Evidence*, also published by Carcanet Press, in 2014.

The book includes re-ordered, revised and updated material from previously published articles:

- Wyatt, S., Harris, A. and Kelly, S. (2016) 'Controversy goes online: Schizophrenia genetics on Wikipedia', *Science and Technology Studies*, vol. 29, no. 1, pp. 13–29.
- Harris, A., Kelly, S. and Wyatt, S. (2014) 'Autobiologies on YouTube: Narratives of direct-to-consumer genetic testing', *New Genetics and Society*, vol. 33, no. 1, pp. 60–78.
- Wyatt, S., Harris, A., Adams, S. and Kelly, S. (2013) 'Illness online: Self-reported data and questions of trust in medical and social research', *Theory, Culture and Society*, vol. 30, no. 4, pp. 128–147.
- Harris, A., Wyatt, S. and Kelly, S. (2013) 'The gift of spit (and the obligation to return it): How consumers of online genetic testing services participate in research', *Information, Communication and Society*, vol. 16, no. 2, pp. 236–257.

- Harris, A., Kelly, S. and Wyatt, S. (2013) 'Counseling customers: Emerging roles for genetic counselors in the direct-to-consumer genetic testing market', *Journal of Genetic Counseling*, vol. 22, no. 2, pp. 277–288.
- Harris, A. (2012) Shopping for a soft sweater and a comfy pair of genes, Book review of *My Beautiful Genome* by Lone Frank. *Genomics, Society and Policy*, vol. 7, pp. 57–64.

Abbreviations and acronyms

ABGC   American Board of Genetic Counseling
ACOG   American Congress of Obstetricians and Gynecologists
AoIR   Association of Internet Researchers
BDNF   brain-derived neurotrophic factor
BRCA   breast cancer susceptibility gene
CDC   Centers for Disease Control and Prevention (US)
CERN   Organisation européenne pour la recherche nucléaire (European Organization for Nuclear Research; originally named Conseil européen pour la recherche nucléaire, from which the acronym was derived)
COMT   catechol-O-methyltransferase
DNA   deoxyribonucleic acid
DTC   direct-to-consumer
DTP   direct-to-provider
FD&C   Food, Drug and Cosmetics Act (US)
FDA   Food and Drug Administration (US)
GWAS   genome-wide association study
HGP   Human Genome Project
KNAW   Koninklijke Nederlandse Akademie van Wetenschappen (Royal Netherlands Academy of Arts and Sciences)
MAOA   monoamine oxidase A
MMR   measles, mumps and rubella
NSGC   National Society for Genetic Counselors (US)
PGP   Personal Genome Project
RCT   randomised clinical trial
RNA   ribonucleic acid
SERT   serotonin transporter
SNP   single nucleotide polymorphism
STS   science and technology studies
UK   United Kingdom
US   United States

1 Introduction

CyberGenetics

It begins with a mucilaginous dollop of spit, the kind of bodily excretion that causes you to heave when you see it on the sidewalk and flinch if a small part hits your cheek when someone speaks. A sample of saliva, so the genetic testing websites claim, will tell you more about yourself than you ever thought you wanted to know.

You first hear about the possibility of buying a genetic test via the internet after scrolling through a newspaper article. Curious, and with some genetic knowledge from undergraduate biology up your sleeve, you order a genetic testing kit from an online company. You find the website, open an account, provide some personal information and enter your credit card details.

Soon the kit arrives and, lying inside a glossy plastic nest, you find a little spittoon. It takes some time to gather the amount of saliva required for analysis (no bubbles allowed). Reading the instructions several times, you mix the specimen with the buffer solution, and screw the cap on tightly. You slip it into a bio-hazard plastic bag and pre-addressed envelope. You complete some paperwork, register online, and drop by your local post office to send the package. Weeks later, when maybe you've forgotten all about it, an email arrives, informing you that your genetic results are ready to view online. You find your password and log in.

Online you find lists of diseases and conditions that you are at an increased, decreased or average risk of contracting in the future, odds calculations, and even a whole series of As, Cs, Ts and Gs (see next section) if you are interested in 'raw' genetic results. You have, with a few clicks and a bit of spit, entered the world of online genetic testing.

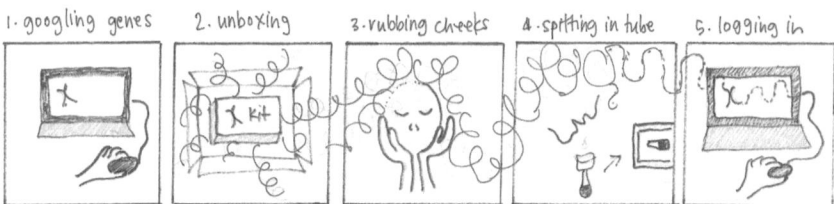

Figure 1.1 Direct-to-consumer genetic testing

Source: Anna Harris

This book critically examines this growing market of direct-to-consumer (DTC) genetic testing from a social science perspective, asking what happens when genetics goes online. Focusing on genetic testing for disease, this book is about the new social arrangements which emerge when genetic testing, a traditionally clinical practice, is taken into different internet spaces. It examines the intersections of new genetics and new media by drawing from three different fields of study: internet studies, the sociology of health and illness, and science and technology studies (STS). Drawing across these fields enables us to understand more about the phenomenon of DTC genetic testing. From internet studies we can learn more about online infrastructures, users' practices and the materiality of virtual exchanges. From science and technology studies we develop insights into the users, the companies, the controversies, the technologies. The sociology of health and illness enriches the other fields with attention to healthcare professionals and practices, and the social life of, and responses to, genetic information.

While there has been a surge of research activity since 2010 concerning DTC genetic testing, particularly in sociology, ethics and law, we believe this is the first book which brings together the social study of genetics and the social study of digital technologies. Not only do we offer a new overview of this emerging field, but we also offer a unique contribution by attending to the digital, and by drawing upon empirical examples from our own research of DTC genetic testing websites, using online and other social research methods (see Appendix A for fuller discussion of our methodological approach). In this book we focus specifically on healthcare genetics. We also offer empirically based insights into themes that resonate with aspects of personalised medicine and other digital genomic futures.

It is often claimed by policy makers, healthcare professionals, the pharmaceutical industry and academic and media commentators that medicine, healthcare, and the wider social meaning and management of health are undergoing major changes. In part this reflects developments in science and technology, which enable new forms of diagnosis, treatment and the delivery of healthcare. It also reflects changes in the locus of care and burden of responsibility for health. Many scientific developments, including genetics and new media, are redefining our understanding of the body, health and disease; at the same time, health is no longer simply the domain of conventional medicine, nor the clinic. The research on which this book is based was conducted largely between the years 2010 and 2012. Given the continued rapid pace of change affecting both genetics and digital technologies, it is therefore important to describe the technologies that were available in that period.

We chose 'cybergenetics' as the main title for the book in order to highlight the ways in which the combination of internet and genetics reconfigures people's experiences of their bodies and data. In light of 'big data' and other developments, DTC genetic testing becomes a way for people to engage with genetic data via technology. 'Cybernetics' was coined in 1948 by Norbert Wiener (1948/1961), an American mathematician best known for his work on the formalisation of feedback mechanisms. He claimed that the emphasis on 'communication and control'

(see section on determinism below) in twentieth-century industrial and other societal practices marked a shift towards treating the body as an integral part of the
information system in terms of incoming and outgoing messages. In the late
twentieth century, with the rise of the internet (see section below about the history
of the internet), the body can be figured as a smart machine that can be digitally
extended and enhanced (Ihde, 2002), expanding upon previous phenomenologi-
cal considerations of human-technology relations. Donna Haraway draws on
cybernetics in her influential work on the cyborg, arguing that rather than reimagining organisms as rigid machines, the concept opens up new possibilities for
recoding our bodies and our selves (Helmreich, 2009). More recently, DTC
genetic testing and measuring and monitoring devices, provide people with information about their genes, and also about their bodies, in a way that certainly
resonates with Wiener's view of cybernetics and Donna Haraway's cyborg, in
which data, technologies, private corporations are internalised in the human body
and neat distinctions between human and machine/technology dissolve. This is
also visualised in Figure 1.1.

To provide context and background for our research, in this Introduction, we
first offer a brief history of the field of DTC genetic testing, in the context of
larger changes in the field of genetics. We then examine the changing role of the
internet in social life, particularly health, and explore intersections between
genetics and the digital. Following this broader discussion, we present the three
main themes of the book: deterministic discourses of genetics and the internet,
and how they connect; the new possibilities for spatial-temporal arrangements
emerging with online genetics; and relations of trust which are continually
performed and negotiated in this field. These three themes thread throughout each
chapter in the book, often mingling in interesting ways, as our analysis of the
DTC genetic testing industry unfolds. The final section in this Introduction
provides a chapter-by-chapter overview of the book, and closes with a poem
about genetics. In the Conclusion, we offer not only another poem but also three
fictional accounts, exploring alternative futures for DTC genetic testing. First, in
Box 1.1, Susan describes her own experiences of being a customer of DTC
genetic testing.

Box 1.1 Autobiology of a direct-to-consumer genetic testing user

Susan Kelly

When we initiated our research, I ordered a 23andMe kit online. The
purpose was to gain insight into the experience of a user of this product, but
it quickly became apparent that this user position gave me insight not only
into the product and interactions surrounding it, but the subjective experience of engaging with the website, the technology, the results and the
process. In short, ordering a 23andMe test gave me more than a window
into 'me' as a particular 'genetic self', but also into the subjective user experiences of how that 'self' is mediated through the product and its interfaces.

We made a decision, based on our ethical approach to using online material, to distinguish 'data' from 'non-data'. The former include publicly available material and my experience of being a 23andMe consumer/user. However, we have not made direct use of material to which I have access in my role as 23andMe consumer; that is contributed by other users with a presumed expectation of privacy. We made this ethical distinction (see also Appendix A) despite the language buried in the 23andMe privacy statement concerning the public nature of some customer-provided information such as postings.

Not at the time a robust social media user nor particularly one of the 'genetically curious', I thought that taking note of my perceptions, decisions and micro as well as overall experience of 23andMe would add to our research. So, unlike some other users we discuss who have attended spit parties or broadcast themselves spitting (see Chapter 2), I spat in the privacy of my office (although I did walk around a bit complaining about how difficult it was to produce so much spit). I filled the tube I received in a brightly covered box (that is still in my office, as I tend to keep boxes in which technological objects arrive), filled out the paperwork and put it in the post.

In this book, traces from my own experience can be found. For example, I know from reading my own results and discussing them at times with others, something about the experience of receiving genetic 'results' by email and trying to make sense of them. I have noted the various communications, updates of consent forms, advertising offers, research updates inviting me to log in to discover whether my genetics accurately predict my preference for savoury or sweet tastes, or the colour of my hair (no, and yes), or other non-life changing 'fun fact' information. I found myself opening some health-related results with trepidation, particularly the results of the few breast cancer-related SNPs (single nucleotide polymorphisms) reported, as I was concerned for my son's future reproductive decisions, although have no known family history of the disease.

I was curious about my own preferences for 'sharing', and whether and when I realised that was what I was doing (quite late in the process, as it turned out). Although professionally curious about consent, I chose to engage with the forms as if I were merely consuming a product, and was dismayed to note how ephemeral was the process and the presentation of the form and its rather important information. I was curious to see how I would respond to the possibility of finding distant relatives in the United States, interested to see how many people invited contact on the basis of a shared haplotype, and found myself profoundly incurious to follow up these potential contacts. (I have a known and well-liked set of first cousins about whom I care far more than these hypothetical distant relatives, although I recognise that this information is very interesting to some people.) I was curious about, although did not report, the 'comment' sections to which I had access, and will say no more about that other than that I am aware that some other users engage very differently than do I.

Raising interesting questions about what my co-author Sally Wyatt has written about 'non-users' (Wyatt, Thomas and Terranova, 2002) and Oudshoorn (2008) about 'selective users', my selectivity was deeply bound up with other aspects of my personality about which I was led to reflect via my engagement with this product. I do not share easily, as might be apparent, and am sceptical of candy-coloured enticements to 'find out more' about myself. My responses to offers to participate in research baffle me. I have spent hours on the telephone answering surveys out of professional empathy, but was not the least interested in merely providing information about whether I would describe myself as cautious or adventurous. I do recognise the appeal of the 'top 10 list' phenomenon used on so many 'news' websites, and am not immune to those (odd where my relationships of trust lie!).

The experience of testing was therefore useful as insight into the online experience, into how I was and was not being engaged by what was presented as possible in the online experience; into which forms of information I found useful or otherwise meaningful, or not; but perhaps most importantly my genetic testing experience gave me insight into what was visible in a casual engagement, and what was not, or less so (what I came to describe as 'pseudo-transparency'). It also caused me to reflect on what kind of a user I am? Am I 'duped', lazy, curious, distractible, trusting or distrusting, entrepreneurial, fearful, working or playing or consuming, ill or healthy?

So, what 23andMe says about me: I have a greater than average risk of deep vein thrombosis (not a surprise given my physiology), have an average or less than average risk of most other diseases, and have a somewhat greater percentage of 'Neanderthal' heritage than is average for someone of my 'ancestry'. I am largely northern European in origin (somewhat interesting given my partially unknown heritage – oops, someone related to me may not want to know that!) and can smell asparagus in my pee. Most of this was not greater insight into 'me', but the test was also wrong in a number of predictions, reducing both my interest and my trust.

It is important for readers of this book to be aware that this form of engagement, of self-reported data, has also informed our analysis. When we talk about trust, when we talk about participation, when we think about the nature of relationships configured or tweaked by the technology, the users, the product, the discourse, as well as the materiality, we are partly informed by this experience of a DTC genetic testing user.

Brief history of direct-to-consumer genetic testing

The Human Genome Project, the much-lauded international effort to decode the entire human genome, was completed in 2003 and an editorial in a leading medical journal welcomed 'the genomic era'; noted for the rise of direct-to-consumer genetic testing (Guttmacher and Collins, 2003). A gene is understood to be the basic physical and functional unit via which traits are transmitted from one generation to the next. Genes consist of specifically ordered sequences of nucleotides at specific positions on a chromosome that code for a specific protein (or in some cases, an RNA molecule). Genes as units of inheritance come in different forms, called alleles. Some diseases are caused by a mutation in one version, or allele, of the gene. Chromosomes are the structures contained in cells into which are bound long strands of deoxyribonucleic acid or (DNA), the molecule that contains the genes or genetic information of all forms of life. The entire complement of genes that code for human beings is contained within 23 chromosomes. Each human being inherits two copies of each chromosome, one from each parent, for a total of 46. The genes contained therein constitute the human genome, which was found via the Human Genome Project, to consist of 20,000–25,000 genes. This meant unravelling the sequences of nucleotides, labelled C (cytosine), G (guanine), T (thymine) and A (adenine) that, in different combinations, are the code containing the information for creating the human form.

The Human Genome Project (HGP) was a 'big science' project, largely publicly funded. One can read about the discovery timeline of the human genome in educational material provided by the Smithsonian Museum in partnership with the National Institutes of Health at a website titled 'Unlocking life's code' (Smithsonian, no date). The timeline travels from the Augustinian friar Gregor Mendel who identified in his famous sweet pea experiments principles of inheritance now known as 'Mendelian', to the beautiful crystallographic photographs of Rosalind Franklin in the 1950s that showed the unique helical structure of DNA, and the Cambridge scientists James Watson and Francis Crick, who modelled the 3D structure of DNA as a 'double helix', also in the 1950s (and was awarded the Nobel Prize), to the mapping of the first genetic diseases in the 1980s (Huntington's disease and cystic fibrosis), to the initiation of the HGP in 1990. The history of genetics, like the history of the DTC genetic testing industry and of the internet, is littered with colourful personalities and fascinating contributions. We consider genetics 'going online' to be another development in this history, with consequences for the further production of information about the human genome, as well as perceptions of its contributions to understanding and intervening in human health.

The public International Human Genome Sequencing Consortium was joined in 1998 by Celera Genomics Corporation, a private company founded by scientist and entrepreneur Craig Ventor. James Watson has since spoken publicly about his opposition to patenting genes (see Gannet, 2014) what some see as the privatisation of a public resource. He has voiced other controversial views with regard to the uses of genetics, and has been labelled by some a eugenicist, sometimes in connection with his open discussion of having a son with the mental disorder schizophrenia and his belief that genetics holds the key for understanding the origins of this condition (*Telegraph*, 2009). The sequencing of the human genome has been characterised as a highly competitive enterprise in which public funding seeded private enterprise, and collaborative data sharing existed in tension with private ownership of data and competition, all of which fuelled rapid leaps of technological capabilities and continue to represent tensions in this arena (see for example, Contreras, 2010).

The 'first draft' of the sequenced human genome was released in 2001, and the project was declared completed in April 2003 (with roughly 99% of the gene-containing regions of the human genome sequenced), an event announced jointly by US president Bill Clinton, UK prime minister Tony Blair (by satellite), Francis Collins (then director of the National Human Genome Project) and Craig Ventor. So much has been written of these events (see for example *Nature*, 2001; Kevles and Hood, 1993; Davies, 2002) that we do not consider it necessary to recount here, but we do want to point to the confluence of public and private, scientific and entrepreneurial interests from which the personal genome industry emerged. For the anonymous 'human' genome, promising translation to vast benefits in human health, quickly became manifest as *personal* genetic testing – the testing of individuals for genes associated with diseases (such as Huntington's disease and cystic fibrosis). These conditions and other traits (such as hair and eye colour, and more controversially, intelligence and athletic ability) are understood to be shared among individuals who have a common genetic heritage (such as families), as different forms of genes encode somewhat different manifestations of traits (known as phenotypes). That is, the general designation 'human genome' quickly became important for what it could tell us about our individuality, what was unique in our combination of alleles, our own genotype, as well as what, on that basis, we might share with others. Yet, searching for genetic origins of some traits that differentiate different groups of people is politically and socially controversial, such as examination of the genetic components of 'race', as is also the search for genetic components of mental disorders (the literatures on these controversies is vast). We examine aspects of controversial science in this book (see Chapter 5), and have focused on genetic tests purporting to identify risks for mental disorders in part because they are scientifically as well as socially controversial. We use various terms to describe the object of this science, including 'psychiatric condition' and 'mental illness', all having different connotations. For example, 'psychiatric condition' is a professional definition, while the terms 'mental disorder' and 'mental illness' are less professionally bounded. 23andMe has also used different terms in different ways in different sites. They use 'mental conditions' on their blog for example, and refer to 'psychiatric disorders' in their research papers.

DTC genetic testing was born from a combination of rapid technological innovation and interest in seeing the translation of fruits of the HGP to medicine and health. Borry and Howard (2008) attribute the rise of DTC genetic testing both to rapid developments in science and the relatively minor presence of genetics in clinical medicine. DTC genetic testing was inaugurated with the launch of Knome in Cambridge, Massachusetts by Harvard Professor of Genetics George Church, which offered whole genome sequencing for $350,000 (Singer, 2007). Church founded the Personal Genome Company in 2005 and has been an outspoken advocate of open access and sharing of genomic data. He is one of a handful of scientists who have publicly sequenced their own genomes (James Watson being the first). Another early entry into the DTC genetic testing industry was deCODE, a company founded in Iceland by Kári Stefánsson and capitalising (controversially) on the genetic and medical information of much of the largely homogeneous Icelandic population (see Fortun, 2008). deCODE was explicitly about the science of genetic discovery. While deCODE logged up years of scientific success, it never turned a profit nor discovered a blockbuster therapy. In 2007, hoping for a new revenue stream, the company introduced deCODEme, offering a US$985 personal genetic test that was part medicine and part recreation. Also in 2007, several other companies entered the personal genome space and began offering genetic testing over the internet, directly to consumers, including 23andMe and Navigenics (see Appendix B for overview of the companies operating in the DTC genetic testing market at the time of our research). These companies hoped 'to usher in a new era of personalised genomic medicine by empowering individuals to access and understand their own genetic information' (23andMe, 2007, cited in McGuire *et al.*, 2009: 3). The saliva-based personal genome kit sold by 23andMe, a company started by Linda Avey, Paul Cusenza and Anne Wojcicki, then-wife of Google founder Sergey Brin, was named 'Invention of the Year' in 2008 by *Time Magazine*. From their initiation, many of these companies advertised the empowerment of consumers to 'know' their own DNA and therefore gain control over their health. The industry has played with a number of ambiguities, including whether the products they sell are medical or recreational, offering information about an individual's genetic ancestry and health-related genetic information, and inviting both playful and health-related motivations from consumers (see Chapter 2). Another ambiguity has concerned the individual genetic information and scientific/biobank aspects of the companies' activities, further capitalising upon both genome sequencing and internet technologies. According to Avey:

> We see ourselves as creating a sort of ecosystem of patients and users. People who stay with us on the website, who keep up with the developments and continue to enter in their data as they gradually get older. Can you see it? These groups – or cohorts – have built-in opportunities for conducting long-term studies that run for years. Studies that you cannot scrape together the money or the research subjects for today.
>
> (Avey, cited in Frank, 2011: 123)

This is an ambitious ethos which is embedded, without being explicit, on the 23andMe website, as the company tried to garner greater involvement in its self-proclaimed 'research revolution'. In a 2010 *Wired* article, Sergey Brin spoke of an accelerated model of research, using Parkinson's disease as an example (Goetz, 2010). 23andMe's moves into the biotechnology industry in 2015 (Harper, 2015) suggest that the assembly of a large database of customers may have been the business strategy all along, and a far more lucrative one than the selling of individual 'personal' genetic testing kits.

While sequencing the human genome has been accompanied by the hope, and promise, that the genetic basis for many complex diseases and traits would soon be identified, this hope has been only partially fulfilled. A great deal of genetic information is now available, while a relatively small number of single gene disorders have been identified; that is, disorders for which defects in a single gene has been identified as the cause (see Chial, 2008). The search for understanding, and more particularly, intervening in human health has more recently turned to increasingly detailed sequencing of entire genomes (or exomes) in large cohorts of individuals in order to identify the multiple genetic contributions to complex conditions. This transition is characterised as the transition from genetics to genomics, from analysis of single genes to that of whole genomes. The DTC genetic testing industry has to a large extent been borne on the wave of genome sequencing, as many tests make use of rapidly advancing sequencing technology.

Playing with these ambiguities and with their novelty, the DTC genetic testing industry has been problematic from both regulatory and market perspectives, most offering tests for the presence of genetic mutations associated with diseases or pathological conditions – from deep vein thrombosis to breast cancer to Alzheimer's disease – and a variety of traits such as ancestry, athleticism, and hair colour. In June 2008, California health regulators sent cease-and-desist letters to Navigenics and twelve other genetic testing firms, including 23andMe. California regulators asked the companies to prove both that a physician was involved in the ordering of each test and that state clinical laboratory licensing requirements were being fulfilled. The controversy sparked a flurry of interest in the relatively new field. In August 2008, Navigenics and 23andMe received state licenses allowing the companies to continue to do business in California.

In late 2013, the US Food and Drug Administration (FDA) sent a warning letter to 23andMe, citing health-related claims on the company's website, and declaring the product in violation of the US Food, Drug and Cosmetics (FD&C) Act. Within five days, a class action lawsuit was filed in the state of California against 23andMe, with the complaints that the information marketed as health-related is not valid or useful, and the additional claim that the same information from customers is contained in databases that were then marketed to the scientific community (Munro, 2013). The company began marketing similar DTC genetic testing products in both Canada and the UK, and, at the time of writing (April 2015), is negotiating with US regulators but not returning health results to new consumers in the US. A message on the 23andMe blog states: 'we remain committed to our mission of empowering individuals with their genetic informa-tion' (23andMe, 2014). It has also announced opening a therapeutic arm with the explicit aim of using the power of its customer numbers and data for novel drug discovery (23andMe, 2015a). deCODEme stopped selling genetic tests via its website in 2013, having declared earlier that it had not turned a profit. In the research upon which this book is based, we have focused primarily, although not exclusively, on 23andMe, as an exemplar of the practices and logics of the DTC genetic testing industry, and the company that has had perhaps the largest impact on cultural imaginations of genomics. While it has been mentioned to us on various occasions that 23andMe is a unique business case, we are convinced that the themes arising from our research have wider resonance in the contemporary study of science and health. (While we focus in this book on health DTC genetic testing products, it is important to note that some companies including 23andMe also include or sell genetic ancestry information products.)

In spite of (or perhaps because of) the intense optimism from scientific supporters, often outspoken in their claims that gene discoveries hold the key to vast improvements in human health, ethicists and social scientists have hewed a more critical line. Both supporters and critics exhibit deterministic echoes. Early identification of genes for serious disorders such as Huntington's disease and breast cancer were critically analysed by many ethicists and social scientists concerned about the potential for such negative outcomes as psychological harm from knowing negative information about one's potential future, or of inadvertently being informed of such information about oneself from a relative or healthcare professional. From these concerns developed a new 'right' – the right 'not to know' one's genetics.

The concept of 'geneticisation' was developed in the late 1980s by Abby Lippman (1991), and was widely adopted among critical observers of genetics. Geneticisation describes 'the ever growing tendency to distinguish people from one another on the basis of genetics; to define most disorders, behaviours, and physiological variations as wholly or partly genetic in origin' (Lippman, 1991: 64). In addition to being widely adopted, the concept has been subjected to a range of critiques, primarily calling for more nuanced recognition of how 'gene for' arguments are deployed by both geneticists and their critics (see, for example, Hedgecoe, 2001). Sociologist Adam Hedgecoe accepts the idea that many of the critics of the 'new' genetics concentrate on the potentially harmful consequences of geneticised understandings of human diseases including mental disorders, and refers to his approach as 'critical bioethics'. As explained in Appendix A about the challenges of studying emergent technological phenomena, we look critically at social science research, including our own, in terms of its role in stabilising the object of its study. In this case, we are reflexive about our attending to the deterministic claims of DTC genetic testing and its cultural impacts, and potentially lending impetus to geneticisation processes. We return to this later in the Introduction, but first we examine another technology that emerged in the latter decades of the twentieth century, namely the internet.

Brief history of the internet and health online

We now turn to the second major protagonist in our book, the internet, and what is often referred to as 'new media' (or digital technologies, computing, information technologies, the web, and increasingly also social media or web 2.0). Digital technologies affect the locus of healthcare, as access to information, diagnosis and treatment move outside the clinical setting (an important aspect of DTC genetic testing), and are increasingly mediated by complex technological infrastructures. Relationships between patients, healthcare professionals, informal care givers, insurance companies and health policy makers are also changing, as people – in their myriad roles – have more opportunities to discuss their experiences of everything from drug reactions to doctors' skills to hospital car parking facilities.

These possibilities are, as we see below, often celebrated as emancipatory (Jenkins, 2006; Surowiecki, 2004; Tapscott and Williams, 2006), by giving people greater access to scientific knowledge and to knowledge about their individual bodies and health, people become empowered to take control of their health. The internet and web 2.0 enable people not only to access information and data but also to generate information and data themselves, in the form of numbers, text, and images. Such data then undergo changes and transformation as they travel from one location to another, from one form to another, and one research context to another. In the case of genetic testing, the focus of this book, people are not only entering phenotypic data about their health on their computer screens they are also providing samples of their DNA. All of these data are converted into digital form so that they can be stored in databases and subsequently analysed by researchers both for the individual and at a collective level.

First, however, we return to the earliest days of the internet. Since its inception in the early 1970s (the exact date is itself subject to dispute), the internet has been embedded in many kinds of scientific endeavour. The internet was initially the preserve of computer scientists, figuring out what it meant to connect computers across distance. It then spread to researchers more generally, and it continues to play an important role in scientific research practice, including the collaborative practices of research groups, the sharing and analysis of large quantities of data, the dissemination of findings, and the social division of research labour (Thomas and Wyatt, 1999; Abbate, 2000; Agar, 2006; Hine, 2006; Leonelli, 2012; Wouters *et al.*, 2013). The internet has affected the nature of scientific questions asked, the interdisciplinary nature of scientific teams, the data sets used and shared, the relationships between those who create and generate data and those who use it, and the distance between researchers and participants. The internet also changes the temporal dimensions of research, with pressure upon scientists to conduct and publish quickly, for media to report findings speedily, and for industry to respond to emerging markets (Nowotny *et al.*, 2001; Pels, 2003). Attention to and investment in research infrastructures, e-science and 'big data' are the most recent manifestations of the importance of digital technologies in scientific research and scholarly practice (Kitchin, 2014; Borgman, 2015).

In the early 1990s, the internet went public, and commercial. The decision of the US National Science Foundation in 1991 to allow commercial traffic on its backbone network (what we now call the internet), and the development of the World Wide Web by Tim Berners-Lee at CERN a few years later, were crucial for the subsequent rapid diffusion of the internet to other countries, industry and individual people. The internet ceased to be the preserve of university-based researchers, and became a medium for the exchange of all sorts of information between all sorts of people and organisations. This opening up of a technology that had previously been the preserve of universities (and, in different technical forms, of banks, large corporations, and state administrations) to people through-out the world led to the first wave of excitement about the social, economic and political possibilities, the dot-com boom of the late 1990s.

People were already using the internet in the late 1990s to find and exchange health-related information. Not only did it provide people with access to medical literature and officially sponsored health websites, people could set up and use a variety of internet-based fora, such as list-servs, bulletin boards, and personal home pages, to share information and personal experiences. These were often celebrated not only by policy makers but also by sociologists for the ways in which they enabled people to become producers of knowledge about health, and to engage in more equal relationships with healthcare professionals (Hardey, 1999; Burrows *et al.*, 2000).

The rise of social media (also referred to as web 2.0, user-generated content, participation, prosumption, and crowd sourcing) in the early years of the twenty-first century made it even easier for people to share information, and made the role of the internet in healthcare practice increasingly visible (Wathen *et al.*, 2008; Adams, 2010). Social media can be defined as web-based applications which facilitate the exchange of ideas and information through their 'architecture of participation' (O'Reilly, 2005). Popular and scholarly accounts of the partici-patory potential of new digital technologies are usually enthusiastic. Twitter, blogs, YouTube, Facebook, and Wikipedia are all lauded for their capacity to harness people's creativity and knowledge, and for their potential to challenge traditional hierarchies in politics, science, and the media. It is claimed these web-based applications have facilitated political uprisings, the solution of scientific problems, and the emergence of hitherto undiscovered talents in music and the arts. Others question the validity of such claims, pointing to the dangers of hoax, misinformation, narcissism, and loss of privacy. Social media are used in areas where citizens and fans have long participated such as politics and popular culture, and in domains where the boundary between expert and amateur is more tightly guarded such as medicine, science, and scholarship. The decentralised architecture of social media and the internet more generally challenges traditional knowledge authorities and hierarchies. Questions arise again, just as they did with web 1.0 in the 1990s, about whether lay inclusion helps to 'democratise' knowl-edge formation or if existing hierarchies are re-enacted online. Just as with genetics, both enthusiasts and critics make use of deterministic arguments (see next section).

Social media have the potential to transform relationships between healthcare professionals, patients, consumers, funding agencies, healthcare systems and industry (Dedding *et al.*, 2011). Notions of 'the clinic' have expanded so that consultations between healthcare professionals and patients are conducted via the internet, using remote monitoring devices and webcams (Christensen and Hickie, 2010; Meropol *et al.*, 2011; Mort, May and Williams, 2003; Oudshoorn, 2012; Pols, 2011). Patient and user group internet fora demonstrate, just as they did in the 1990s, that the internet can be a space to share experiences and resources, discuss research developments and act as a platform for (mediated) exchange between users (Kaplan *et al.*, 2011), but now with more audio-visual options. Patient-experience websites such as HealthTalkOnline and PatientsLikeMe demonstrate other ways in which patients, carers and others, can engage with each other, and potentially conduct their own research (Allison, 2009).

In making use of these possibilities, people are generating enormous amounts of transactional data while going about their everyday (online) activities, as already described in the preceding section. Such data are of enormous value not only to biomedical and market researchers but also to scholars in the humanities and social sciences (Savage and Burrows, 2007). This is particularly evident in healthcare, where information about people's states of health and illness is now easily amassed digitally, for research and other purposes, through a range of technological artefacts and practices (Foster and Young, 2012; Fearnley, 2006; Oudshoorn, 2011; Pols, 2011; Ginsberg *et al.*, 2009). Digital technologies facilitate not only more detailed measurement and monitoring (such as the 'quantified self' movement, see Lupton, 2012) but also the diffusion of responsibility for providing data from medical researchers to individual citizens, who are considered to be particularly helpful in generating 'zettabytes of medical data' (Swan *et al.*, 2010). Individuals are encouraged to become more actively involved in data collection because they are considered to be the best (yet often 'untapped') resource for information about their own states of health and illness.

In this book, we focus on different types of internet-based platforms. The most prominent are the websites of companies selling direct-to-consumer genetic tests. Such sites are no longer the 'flat' sites, common in the mid-1990s, which were often little more than online brochures and leaflets. Many of the DTC genetic testing companies use a variety of web 2.0 platforms in order to engage and interact with consumers, including blogs, Twitter and YouTube. User-generated content such as feedback on forums and blog comments feed into company research design. Users' web activity is also collected through log files and cookies, so that web behaviour data are used by the companies in order to monitor use of their website, to improve their services and to tailor and customise content for customers. Data are also exchanged when people purchase genetic tests, as we describe more fully in the section below about trust in both online spaces and in genetics.

In later chapters, we also examine YouTube, a very popular example of social media. YouTube was launched in 2005 as a user-friendly video-sharing site, and was bought by Google in 2006 (Shifman, 2012: 189). It has been described as enabling a new visual genre of individual expression, with some scholars also referring to a YouTube community (Shifman, 2012; Wesch, 2008). It is a particularly good place in which to examine stories about genetic testing for a number of reasons. First, it is used by many DTC genetic testing companies, and presumably by a number of their customers as well. Second, it provides access to users' stories in the public domain, with qualitatively rich details about the process of undergoing testing and interpreting results, results which are their own rather than hypothetical scenarios. And finally, it is a website, just like the genetic testing websites, where the individual meets the collective, where individual stories and genetic data are shared and discussed and the private is rendered public. Elsewhere, but not included in this book, we have also examined English-language Wikipedia pages as a source of information about schizophrenia, and considered their role not only in the representation of knowledge but also in knowledge production (Wyatt, Harris and Kelly, 2016).

The internet continues to be celebrated as a tool of empowerment, particularly in the scientific and medical fields. But the various forms of internet-mediated healthcare raise issues concerning privacy, expertise, access, exclusion and hypochondria/anxiety. Others have shown that web architecture and engagement with web technologies are more complex, involving the replication of dominant hierarchies, and possibly the introduction of new forms of inequality and exploitation (Goldberg, 2011; König, 2013; Proulx *et al.*, 2011; Terranova, 2000). For example, in relation to Wikipedia, Niederer and van Dijck (2010) suggest that many discussions have been misguided in that they focus on the people involved, neglecting the technological tools and managerial dynamics that structure and maintain content. In this book, we build upon these critical studies of the internet, and we recognise the sometimes contradictory aspects of web engagement, where internet infrastructure both enables and constrains engagement with scientific research (the methodological implications of this are discussed more fully in Appendix A).

In the early days of networked personal computers, users often needed techni-cal expertise in order to make the technology work. But more than twenty years later, the public and commercial internet is well on the way to becoming black boxed, as the inner workings of computers and the means for connecting them are increasingly taken for granted, at least in some parts of the world. This only makes it more crucial to pay attention to how the internet affects how patients, carers, commercial organisations, scientists and medical professionals under-stand, interpret and engage with science and other forms of knowledge. In this book we examine how the architecture of the internet reconfigures and makes visible relationships and flows of data and information between consumers, patients, healthcare professionals, scientists, and private companies. By recognis-ing that different platforms can and may be used differently by actors, providing different kinds of health-related information, such an analysis aims to keep the black box open.

Having introduced the two main protagonists of our book – genetics and the internet – in the remainder of this Introduction, we outline the three main themes which weave through the following chapters. These have already been alluded to and they are determinism, both genetic and technological, changing spatial-temporal relations of healthcare, and trust.

Intersecting determinisms: when genetic testing goes online

The preceding two sections demonstrate the long-standing belief that techno-scientific progress equals broader social progress. Discussions around genetics are often characterised by 'genetic determinism', however contested such determinism remains in understanding human health and behaviour. The internet is also subject to similar claims, appealing to the transformative power of the technology, whether it is the Twitter revolution in any of a number of countries, or a revolution in healthcare, such as that promised by personalised medicine, and announced by EU commissioner Neelie Kroes. In March 2104, Kroes delivered a perfect example of this, in a speech about 'mHealth', about the possibilities for mobile technologies to help citizens 'control their care' and also as a benefit for governments dealing with ageing populations, and an enormous business opportunity for European hardware and software companies (Kroes, 2014). Naming epochs according to the techno-sciences of their times is a form of technological determinism characteristic of the twentieth and twenty-first centuries, a 'habit of thought and language of associating places and times with their technologies … even if causality is not always explicit' (Wyatt, 2008: 168).

In this book, we explore this intersection of determinisms, where two of the alleged 'epoch-defining' technologies of the twenty-first century come together in the form of online DTC genetic testing. Genetic and digital determinisms are deeply interwoven not only in the products and product claims but also in the representations of uses and users that are at the heart of DTC genetic testing. Certainty results when genetically deterministic thinking is enabled by the medium of the internet. One of our contentions is that the value of DTC genetic testing lies in no small part in its appeal to a 'gene for …' (eye colour/diabetes/Alzheimer's disease/schizophrenia/violence – delete as appropriate) understanding of the relationship between genetics and human health and illness.

We are interested in exploring this intersection as a form of convergence, in the sense of mutually enabling discourses about and embedded in technologies. Specifically, we explore how deterministic thinking is embedded within genetic science, and the selling of genetic testing products to consumers online. We refer to these as 'intersecting determinisms', with implications not only for governance but for the ways in which we study such new products and phenomena (see also Appendix A). Our assumption is that determinisms of genetics are converging with determinisms of the internet, and from this convergence, genetic testing products have been developed, with internet-enabled reach directly to potential consumers and research participants far beyond the clinic.

We examine these determinisms symmetrically. In other words, we do not take one form of determinism or another to be 'true' but rather we examine them 'in the making', as deterministic discourses are contradicted, subverted and negotiated in complicated ways as individuals, healthcare professionals, companies and regulators, constantly weave together social and technological practices. We also recognise multiple determinisms. In earlier work, one of us distinguished between four types of technological determinism: normative needs, descriptive, justificatory, and methodological (Wyatt, 2008). Each of these is discussed below, as they relate to DTC genetic testing, and our own approach to studying this phenomenon.

At the beginning of this section, we provided instances of normative technological determinism, when genetics and the internet become so embedded in everyday life that they become taken for granted in public discourses. The digital or information age is driven by the internet, which has relatively quickly become an integral part of the everyday activities of individuals, science, and business. As we saw in the previous sections about genetics and the internet, there are many platforms upon which health service users, clinicians, scientists and other interested parties can share data and information about genetics and genetic tests, incorporating modern science into centuries of understanding of inheritance, and using this to make sweeping generalisations about the nature of health, illness and humanity. For example, genetic causality for mental illness has been argued to have the potential to alleviate stigma and guilt, as well as lead to significant distress. Emily Martin (2007) suggests that belief in a genetic component of bipolar disorder gives those suffering from the disease some hope that in the future there will be treatment based on scientific knowledge. The anthropologist herself found comfort in the fact that her problems were not entirely within her control.

Descriptive technological determinism can be found in the everyday accounts provided by users engaging in DTC genetic testing, as we saw in the description of doing the test and receiving the results that opened this chapter. As we see in the next chapter, users sometimes post videos of themselves on YouTube, sometimes doing the test and sometimes opening their test results for the first time. We find, consistent with the research of others (Lock *et al.*, 2006; Cox and McKellin, 1999; Dingel *et al.*, 2015), that people have various different 'tracks' for explaining genetic links to illness and that one of these tracks is generally highly deterministic, while others are marked by uncertainty, with individuals constantly switching between tracks. Forums administered by genetic testing companies and other websites we have examined also reflect this switching between genetic deterministic descriptions and narratives. Some of those posting on fora refer to themselves by their alleles, and other understandings of health and illness. In Chapters 2 and 5 we discuss further how the internet becomes an infrastructure which not only structures and constrains these kinds of exchanges and engagement with genetics, but at the same time allows individuals to use internet platforms in creative ways.

Justificatory technological determinism can be found most obviously in the marketing and selling of genetic tests. But it is also implicitly embedded in the concerns expressed by many members and organisations within scientific and medical communities regarding the risks such information may have for individuals, who may misunderstand and misinterpret genetic information. For example, in relation to the first, 23andMe described schizophrenia in 2012 as 'highly heritable'. There is no mention on the website that only a small part of the heritability of schizophrenia has been studied genetically, and that most remains unexamined in terms of the influence of non-genetic effects. The sample schizophrenia report for the fictitious Mr Mendel offered by 23andMe implies that they test for two proposed markers of the disease, with summaries and hyperlinks to relevant scientific studies, studies which were conducted in specific populations and which have not been replicated. Many of the companies we examined mobilised genetic determinism in order to market their product, reinforced by the supporting commentaries and links to scientific studies, the complexities of which are not discussed on the company websites. The companies deploy this genetic deterministic discourse in order to justify the purchase of their tests. Consequently, the companies reinforce a degree of certainty and give the impression of stable facts, deliberately reducing complexity through their selective and strategic use of genetic markers and scientific resources. Justificatory technological determinism is not only built into the company's products and product claims but also by many who want to control testing. Objections to the test by healthcare professionals and organisations are underscored by the attitude that the genetic test will change how individuals think about and behave toward their health, and that this information is inaccurate, so they should not have access to such tests.

Distinguishing between normative, descriptive and justificatory forms of technological determinism helps us to understand how genetics and digital technologies combine in the offering of DTC genetic testing. Methodological determinism, however, is the most important for us as researchers, in order to understand our own relationship with our object of study. By taking technologies as the starting point of our analysis, it could be argued that our research question is already technologically deterministic, that we are partaking in a form of methodological technological determinism, a kind of determinism practised by many STS scholars who study technologies. Even as we critique deterministic accounts, we must recognise that by placing science and technology at the centre of our accounts, we may also be guilty of technological determinism.

While doing the research on which this book is based, we constantly considered the methodological challenges posed by studying a topic that was novel, emergent, and controversial. In particular, we were concerned with the problematic of stabilising an object of inquiry by studying it, conferring it with more stability as an object than it ontologically possesses, and also contributing to the justificatory determinism and hype surrounding it (Woolgar, 2002). Another challenge has been the recognition that the science, the technologies, the companies and products themselves are moving targets, responding to their environment, including regulators, academic critics and consumers. In other words, the object of DTC genetic testing is itself reflexive. For example, following criticism that genetic tests should be accompanied by counselling, 23andMe added a link to an online commercial genetic counselling company with counsellors trained in the 23andMe product (see Chapter 3). As discussed above, the 2013 FDA ruling had direct consequences not only for the commercial but also for the research activities of the company.

Of course, many social science researchers have already shown that individuals engage with genetic information in complex ways. Such research tends to debunk claims and fears of genetic determinism, revealing the mundane, idiosyncratic and rather undramatic ways in which individuals interpret and include genetic information into their own sense of personhood and understandings of disease and illness (e.g. Lock *et al.*, 2006; Cox and McKellin, 1999), and as we discuss in the next chapter when we introduce the concept of 'autobiology'. Such work moves the social study of genetics beyond simple deterministic arguments.

But deterministic arguments remain, in the ways companies market genetic testing (normative and justificatory), how professional and lay users talk about it (normative, justificatory, descriptive), and how we as researchers may use it in our own research designs (methodological).

It is not difficult to critique the ways in which companies use determinism to sell their products, be they genetic tests or smart watches, or doctors and privacy campaigners who use it to demand tighter regulation, but we also need to recognise that some degree of determinism does describe really quite well how different actors understand and articulate their interpretation of the effects of technology on their lives. There is much important social science research that moves beyond deterministic arguments by highlighting the complex ways in which individuals engage with genetic and digital technologies (Lee *et al.*, 2013; Lupton, 2012; Pálsson, 2009; Prainsack, 2011; Tutton, 2014). In this section, we have drawn attention to the genetic and other determinisms that are still present, in the naming of epochs, in the ways in which genetic testing and information technology companies market their products, in the reasons that regulatory organisations give for their attempts to control the genetics and information technology industries, and in the ways in which people describe their relationships to genetic and digital technologies. We have also used this discussion to reflect on our own analysis of DTC genetic testing.

As scholars we need to take technological determinism seriously. As Wyatt (2008) has argued, we need to treat actors' own identifications and interests symmetrically with analysts' identifications and interests. We cannot simply ignore technological determinism because we find it inadequate as an explanation. It is all around us, especially in relation to both genetics and digital technologies, so we need to pay attention to it.

There are many possible readings of the deterministic narratives circulating in the media, online, and in the material produced by companies involved in genetic testing. In the following chapters, we pay close attention to the determinisms in contemporary society, and to our own use of them, in order to understand more fully the complex dynamics of sociotechnical developments wrapped up with genetics, the internet and other technologies.

New spaces for health-e relations?

As described earlier in this chapter, the internet opens up new possibilities for people to locate health-related information, and new spatial-temporal relations among patients/consumers, healthcare professionals, and creators and holders of biological information (public or private, industry or otherwise). This leads us to ask, what happens when genetics goes online? What new spatial-temporal relationships are made possible, how are they framed, represented and understood, and how can we study them? In terms of spatial-temporal relations, what are we to make of the disparately located forms of work, agency and engagement involved in DTC genetic testing, with spitting and receiving of interpretations of personal genetic data occurring in bedrooms or other non-clinical locations; spit and data processing occurring in diverse locations; and counselling offered (if at all) as an electronically mediated communication between two individuals unknown to each other? We argue that the DTC genetic testing industry opens up possibilities in terms of the spatial–temporal spaces that have the potential to reconfigure social relations around emerging healthcare technologies, and particularly between professionals and others.

As soon as the DTC genetic testing industry caught the attention of ethicists, social scientists and legal observers, questions have been raised about ways in which healthcare professionals are involved. Concerns have focused primarily on the lack of mediation of complex genetic information by professionals with expertise in the interpretation of health-related genetics. Genetic information, as we have seen, had already been identified as potentially harmful, as well as being based on complex science requiring interpretation to be meaningful to individuals concerned about health risks. There is a darker history to the idea that genetic information is potentially harmful, one that invites analysis of another ambiguity within the DTC genetic testing industry, that between individual autonomy and expert (largely medical) control of information. Clinical genetics, in some countries supported by the profession of genetic counselling, has developed since around the 1900s, as a mediator of genetic science to the public (although genetics in public health has a much longer history). This history involved public health 'ownership' of genetics (e.g. Paul, 1998; Kerr and Shakespeare, 2002) and has included public health campaigns to use genetic knowledge – or at least knowledge of heredity – to intervene in reproduction in order to improve population health.

Genetic counselling is a term coined in the US in the 1940s by Dr Sheldon C Reed (Veatch, LeRoy and Bartels, 2003). With this development, clinical genetics took ownership of the practice of genetic counselling, and initiated an ethos of individual autonomy; that is, that individuals should decide for themselves how to manage their genetic risks, particularly with regard to reproduction. The American Society of Human Genetics published a definition of genetic counselling in 1975 (Veatch *et al.*, 2003). This definition emphasised that genetic counselling is a process of communication and included patient autonomy as an important element. Thus, from the last century, both the right to make decisions about one's own genetic risks and a perhaps paternalistic control of the process of interpretation of genetic information by the medical profession have characterised social relations around genetic information. A further set of social relations includes those between the producers and users of genomic knowledge. However, one of the selling points of the DTC genetic testing industry has been the empowerment accompanying direct access to one's own genome, as part of a broader ethos of 'citizen science', which would allow individuals to go beyond autonomy within the traditional patient/physician relationship and, so empowered, to 'take charge' of their own health and futures. Sandra Lee has recently discussed this point in terms of potentiality: 'The marketing and consumption of personal genetic information relies on constructions of biological potential that result from struggles over the ability to control and act on individualized genetic information and to translate it into meaning' (Lee, 2015: S77).

In marketing statements such as 'By knowing more about your DNA, you may be able to take steps towards living a healthier life' (23andMe, 2015b), it appears that the DTC genetic testing industry is allying itself to emerging notions of rights, citizenship, and what we might term 'biological ownership', meaning notions of control over personal information including the biological (such as DNA-containing spit), health outcomes data, and lifestyle choices. This shift has been identified by some observers as in line with the 'new public health' in which responsibility for health (largely in the form of making healthy life choices, but extending to knowledge of one's health-related data) falls upon individual citizens rather than the state (e.g. Peterson and Lupton, 1996; Lemire, Sicotte and Paré, 2008).

We return to these issues in the notion of the 'dispersed subject' discussed in the Conclusion, Chapter 6. The DTC genetic testing industry has taken note of criticisms concerning unmediated access to genetic information and responded in a number of ways, including re-configuring relationships on offer between consumers and healthcare professionals. Companies now provide a range of relationships with medical professionals, from staffing physicians to order tests, to offering genetic counselling either directly or as an add-on service, to affiliating with online commercial genetic counselling services, to claiming their products do not offer medical diagnostic information but are for educational or recreational purposes only. McGowan, Fishman and Lambrix (2010) have referred to some of these relationships as direct-to-provider (DTP) marketing strategies and have examined how these services are provided, particularly in terms of expertise. A survey by McGuire *et al.* (2009) of social media users, some percentage of whom had purchased tests, found that 60 per cent of respondents who had used the services considered the results to be medically diagnostic, and a full 78 per cent of all respondents would ask their physicians to help interpret results. While we cannot find evidence that this potential flood of personal genomic information has landed on healthcare professionals in a large way, we do argue that the DTC genetic testing industry has the potential to, if not reconfigure, at least open new spaces for social relationships around genomic and more broadly medical expertise, and for expert/lay relations.

While acknowledging that this is a broader phenomenon, as an exemplar, we have explored spatial-temporal relations involving genetic counselling in some depth (see Chapter 3). We find, and argue, that in moving online, genetic counselling has altered some of the core tenets of the discipline (for example, considering the family unit with regard to genetic information rather than only the individual). Further, as Kate O'Riordan correctly notes, DTC genetic tests are more than merely biomedical in the relationships they entangle, as they operate 'at the intersection of digital biosociality, consumption and knowledge production' (O'Riordan, 2013: 518). As such, they open spaces for social relationships around identity, sociality, economics, and the politics of knowledge that we explore in this volume. In this vein, we argue that the spaces opened for emerging social relations suggest the emergence of more playful forms of engagement with biomedical science and the potential futures they portend via personal genomics, playfulness we capture in the concept of 'autobiologies' (see Chapter 2), and playfulness that is itself enrolled in the marketing and product displays of companies including 23andMe, which market personal genomics as not only self-knowledge, but material for playful self-creation, extension and representation.

While we question, as do others, the complexities and usefulness of genetic information provided by DTC genetic testing (e.g. US Federal Trade Commission, 2006; Hunter *et al.*, 2008), we choose here to reflect on the problematics of social relationships opened by DTC genetic testing spaces including those between commercial and medical fields, and issues raised by internet technologies being used in telegenetic and other quasi-clinical settings. The ways in which the DTC genetic testing industry has responded to such critiques reminds us that as an object of study it is a moving target, a reflexive object of multiple critical gazes (an issue we explore in more depth in Appendix A about the methods we have used).

We also ask what these potentially reconfigured relationships mean for consumers/patients, and suggest that our understanding of users, the forms of subject/ivities engendered, and the social relationships in which they engage, are fluid and dynamic, a challenge indeed for researchers trying to examine such phenomena (see also Chapter 2 and Appendix A).

Changing relations of trust: in bodies, expertise, science and technology

When genetics goes online, trust becomes an important aspect of how these different relations between users, healthcare providers, industry and governing bodies that we have outlined are assembled and reconfigured. Already issues of health, especially the lack of it, raise many questions about trust: in one's body and its responses; in individual healthcare professionals and informal care givers; in medical knowledge; and in healthcare systems. Digital technologies affect all of these, as we have discussed earlier in this chapter. Online DTC genetic testing is a powerful example of the ways in which digital technologies reconfigure trust relationships concerning health and illness, between people, their bodies, and experiential knowledge. We work on the premise that issues of trust are brought into relief wherever there are perceived to be exchanges of information, or the possibility of its appropriation. The most obvious exchange in DTC genetic testing concerns how individuals send a sample of their saliva or cheek swab to an internet-based company in order to receive genetic information about themselves. Information is also exchanged in the purchase of genetic tests through customers' provision of personal information such as financial details, online account information, and through their potential ongoing engagement on the site through commenting on fora or blogs.

The type of data being shared by consumers includes words and numbers as well as something visceral, as they provide bodily material that is analysed. As we discussed earlier, information is returned to the customer in the form of raw genetic test results, analysis and interpretation of genetic data, and material on the website, blogs and fora about genetics, genetic testing and other company activities. Information is also shared between users, as they can openly invite or search for others to view their genetic results, and through the user-generated content on various platforms. 23andMe asks its customers to provide further information about their health, personal traits and behaviour via simple online surveys. The information gathered is linked to the customer's genetic data and contributes toward building a research repository of genetic and health information to be used by researchers and other third parties such as researchers and pharmaceutical companies.

Throughout this book we explore the different kinds of trust relationships entangled in online genetics. There are four main kinds of trust we examine closely:

- trust in genetics;
- trust in the internet;
- trust in companies; and
- trust in research and research data.

We have already discussed how online genetics is built upon the basis that genetic information can tell people something important about their past, present and future. In buying a genetic test, the customer is implicitly demonstrating some trust in the genetic basis of health conditions and human traits. Companies foster the geneticisation of health and behaviour on their websites, although acknowledging in relatively small print the 'influence' of environmental and other factors. In many ways public trust in the scientific research process is arguably fragile after the wake of highly publicised scandals such as the MMR vaccine link to autism and instances of research fraud. Greater public participation in science is viewed by many as a way to enhance public trust in scientific knowledge. These trust relations are complex and certainly the kinds of trust being played out in the context of online genetic testing are not straightforward. Anthropologists (e.g. Lock *et al.*, 2006) have argued that rather than strengthening beliefs about the genetic basis of life processes, genetic testing is interpreted in the context of existing notions of family inheritance. While many of these researchers have not looked at trust specifically, we can extrapolate that, like other forms of health information, genetic information that is most consistent with pre-existing expectations about heritable characteristics and diseases is generally perceived as more trustworthy. We explore this theme more fully when we examine the ways that users engage with interpretation of their tests in Chapter 2.

Trust in digital technologies, particularly the internet, is another form of trust embedded in the online genetic testing process. Sites with identifiable commercial interests have to put significant effort into communicating trust. On genetic testing websites, emphasis is given to the security of their website as a place to share sensitive information, including genetic, health and financial details, with privacy highlighted. In privacy statements, there are technical details about firewalls, secure online payment systems, genetic information and health information being kept separate from account information, encryption of data and connections, monitoring of employees' use of databases, and restricted access to internal servers and data centres. The online genetic testing market presents the internet as a relatively risk-free place in which to find out genetic information about yourself, information that is not necessarily tied to your medical record. In regards to sharing information on the internet, the companies promote and attempt to normalise this activity. Sharing genetic information is encouraged among users, in order to find relatives or others with similar genetics. This also includes sharing further information about health and other behaviours for research purposes, as we explore in more detail in Chapter 4. The internet is viewed as a way in which to democratise genetic knowledge, and empower users to do what they want with this information. The internet is promised to be a platform by which consumers or participants can be freed from institutional power and actively engaged in finding out more about their genetic selves.

While the DTC genetic testing market is premised on some kind of relations of trust concerning genetics and the internet, each company also needs to foster trust in its own product. The companies have different ways of doing this. Links to trustworthy institutions are made through the promotion of recent funding by the National Institute of Health, profiles of scientific advisory boards members with details of university affiliations, and hyperlinks to the National Society of Genetic Counsellors and independent genetic counselling services. We examine these complicated relationships of trust with healthcare providers, particularly genetic counsellors, in Chapter 3. Public trustworthiness in the DTC genetic testing enterprise is also achieved through promotion of the companies in various media outlets such as newspaper and TV, with celebrity endorsement by well-known personalities such as Oprah Winfrey.

As we have already outlined, an important part of the business model for several DTC genetic testing companies is the database of information that they build on users, containing not only their genetic testing results but also the information provided through online surveys. This database is used and promoted as an important tool in conducting cutting-edge scientific research on the genetic basis of health conditions. It is important that companies such as 23andMe, a leader in this field, establish relations of trust with their customer base in order to conduct research, as well as trusting their customers, for the research differs from more traditional medical research in a number of ways, particularly in the use of self-reported data.

Typically, genetic researchers rely on medical records for health information, or on data collected directly by medical researchers. The research conducted by 23andMe, however, relies on information provided by its customers/medical subjects/citizen researchers/biosubjects/guinea pigs. Self-reported data is used not only by genetic testing companies such as 23andMe but also by an increasing number of online non-profit health organisations such as PatientsLikeMe (Allison, 2009; Wicks *et al.*, 2011) and others (e.g. the Personal Genome Project, Genomera, TuAnalyze and LAMsight), as well as in state-run databases (e.g. the Icelandic Biobank). The use of self-reported data blurs and contests the boundaries of expertise previously established in the medical research world. Self-reported data acknowledge lay knowledge about one's body and healthcare experiences, yet are often criticised by scientific and medical researchers who believe they are unreliable (Arnquist, 2009; Prainsack, 2011). By showing trust in self-reported data, in the individual as a source of information about their own health behaviour, rather than the medical record produced by clinicians, these practices foster new ways of thinking about the relations of trust between research participants and researchers. While the company trusts self-reported data, although it recognises that the data might be 'incomplete', or 'dirty'. As individuals have personal and familial health narratives that are not necessarily 'accurate' in a scientific or medical sense (see Chapter 2), this raises interesting questions about the health information supplied. This model of research is based on the premise that any errors that do occur are outweighed by the significant number of participants in the study.

In order to foster participation in this research model, the company needs to build upon the trust relations they have established with the customer through the purchase of the test. The company also needs to build trust into their research paradigm in order for customers to share further personal information through the answering of the surveys. This is done through building trust in their research process and through public engagement and the early feedback of research results to participants and would-be participants using various platforms such as blogs, fora and Twitter. This is something currently encouraged in medical research, but as yet under-realised. The stabilisation of controversy, whether this means controversial research techniques or disputes over the genetic basis of disease for example, is also another way in which to build trust, something which we explore in more detail in Chapter 5. Finally, there are attempts to foster trust by allowing participants and customers to communicate with the company via social media, enabling the company can react quickly to areas of distrust.

Establishing relations of trust with consumers/participants is an important aspect of online genetic company research however, in order to have the infrastructural arrangements to conduct this research, companies rely on venture capital and a trusting relationship with investors. Funders want to see a return for their investment, and it increasingly appears as if profits will not be obtained from the sale of genetic tests, but rather from the potential of the research database to generate revenue from pharmaceutical companies, other biotechnology firms, and through the development of patents. In order to secure these profits however, companies potentially jeopardise trust relations with consumers. The online genetic testing market is one in which the main players must carefully balance profits and participation, an ever more precarious balancing act. As internet users become increasingly aware of the business practices behind sites (e.g. in the highly-publicised dispute about properly informing customers about privacy policies and settings on the social networking site Facebook), maintaining trust amid growing consumer scepticism (e.g. through information strategies that demonstrate transparency in practice) will remain important.

In summary, trust relations are integral to online genetics. Trust is not an inherent property of the sites and is not automatic on the part of anyone visiting the sites. Trust is tied into a whole system of interactions – interpersonal, discursive, physical and technical. These relations need to be built into the internet transactions, and draw upon broader trust relations such as trust in the internet and trust in genetics. In many ways, these issues are neither new nor specific to web 2.0 and/or the health domain. Issues related to ethics, trust, representativeness, online identity, and so on have been raised since researchers began studying the web in the mid-1990s. But the web and associated research opportunities continue to grow and change, which may lead to new issues, new iterations of old issues or changes in the nature and scale of existing issues. Research models such as that adopted by 23andMe, for example, introduce new kinds of trust relations into the sharing of information on the internet, relations which involve the sharing of both numerical and textual data as well as bodily material. Whether this web-based model of conducting research will increase public trust in genetic research, and medical research more broadly remains to be seen. The online genetics industry may be fostering new kinds of relations of trust between research participants and researchers by showing trust in self-reported data, in the individual as a source of information about their own health behaviour, rather than the medical record, and sharing results so quickly with participants.

Again, as will become evident throughout this book, such relations are not so straightforward. As they expand their customer base, commercial companies such as 23andMe are building a powerful research resource for their own purposes, which are attractive to third party researchers and other commercial enterprises. It therefore remains integral to our understandings of how not only genetic testing but also health and illness play out online and in these commercial contexts, by remaining attentive to how relations of trust are built, rebuilt, assembled and configured between different actors, mindful of how this is affected by the digital. The trust relationships between actors from science, industry and the public, themselves often mediated via the internet, are fragile and unstable. This is especially true when the science (genetics), and the means of data collection (self-reported data via the internet) are themselves emerging.

Overview of book

Throughout the book we return to the main themes discussed above: deterministic discourses of genetics and the internet, the new possibilities for spatial-temporal arrangements emerging with online genetics; and relations of trust in this field. Chapters 2 and 3 focus on two important groups of human actors, users of DTC genetic testing, and genetic counsellors, as an example of healthcare professionals implicated in this new market.

Chapter 2 introduces readers to users of DTC genetic testing, looking specifically at a celebrity genetic testing user who has written an autobiography on genetics and 'non-celebrity' users who post videos about testing on YouTube. We analyse these stories as autobiologies, the study of and story about one's own organism. This is positioned within the literature about 'patients in waiting', arguing that autobiologies are told in the context of encounters with one's own biology that are being reconfigured with the introduction of new technologies.

In Chapter 3, we examine how the healthcare profession of genetic counselling has been represented on DTC genetic testing websites, blogs and other online material. We focus on genetic counselling because it is a healthcare profession that has developed specifically to inform and counsel patients about the meaning of genetic testing and its results for patients and their relatives. DTC genetic testing can be seen to challenge many of the traditional roles of counsellors, and to provide opportunities for new ones. Five overlapping roles are presented: genetics educator, mediator, lifestyle/health adviser, risk interpreter, and entrepreneur.

Chapter 4 returns to the users, but in their role as 'research participants'. DTC genetic testing is at the forefront of this development and in this chapter we examine the kinds of "participatory" practices which genetic testing consumers are enticed to engage in, particularly how are being enrolled into research. We consider how these participation practices are paradoxical in terms of their potential to be both alienating and emancipatory. In critically examining the broader cultural processes at work we focus on the economic underpinnings of online participation and the free labour of participants.

DTC genetic testing is itself a controversial practice, and schizophrenia genetics is a highly contested area of science in which genetics has long played an inconclusive role. In Chapter 5, we examine how DTC genetic testing companies represent and make use of controversial scientific claims. We find that scientific resources are used across different platforms, strategically, to present a stabilised version of schizophrenia genetics; and in a more nuanced way, on the blogs of the same genetic testing companies, to present a more uncertain (although always hopeful) representation of science.

We conclude with speculative fictional imaginaries of our cybergenetic futures in poetry, letters, a newspaper article and future archaeology report. These fictions reflect on the possibilities for a world where genetics not only goes online but where digital technologies and scientific knowledges are becoming ever more intertwined, opening new spaces for relations between technology users, bodies and commercial companies; reshaping meanings of trust and participation; and shifting identities and roles and places of interaction.

This book is based on original research conducted by the authors (see acknowledgements), but for ease of reading, we have kept methodological details to a minimum. But methodology is important, and some readers will be interested to know more about how we collected material, especially as conducting research about emerging phenomena presents particular challenges. In Appendix A we summarise the range of methods used throughout the book, including a chapter-by-chapter guide of the methodological choices made. We examine the ethics of doing research, particularly when using web-based methods and data. The ontological implications of our methodological choices, the ways in which methods bring objects of research into being, are explored. We also reflect upon the epistemological implications of our methodological choices. Even though we do not claim to offer a 'how to' guide, Appendix A offers seven principles for doing research about emergent techno-scientific phenomena.

This chapter closes with a poem written by Caoilinn Hughes, reflecting upon genetics and labour, the material production and destinations of knowledge, the seeds of determinism, and the uncertainties of 'potentiality'. Hughes's poem captures many of the themes we examine in this book, as well as presaging the turn to imagination in the writing we present in the conclusion of the book, where via speculative fictional imaginaries of cybergenetic futures we suggest an alternative exploration of the book's themes. As presented in the seven principles for doing research about emergent technoscience, we appeal to playful and imaginative speculations about futures.

Apple falls from the tree

after Gregor Johann Mendel (1822–1884)

by Caoilinn Hughes

I

Place in two untiring hands as many hectares of monastery garden;
breed, mongrelize, tally, catalogue with obedience, self-discipline,
three dozen pea species; cultivate the principles of heredity.

Take the Liturgy of the Hours literally. Blot out all noise of Darwin,
for Goodnesse sake. Feed in silence at grave refectory tables; forgo
     tonguing
pea jackets from your teeth. Later, if you must, you may mutter

over careful protein register: round or wrinkled ripe seed shape;
green or yellow endosperm; white or purple petal colour; pods pinched
or ballooned; dwarfed or drawn-out stem; flower position axial or terminal.

Kneel in your tunic, cincture; stoop in hooded shoulder. Produce the effect
of labouring for the Kingdom of Heaven. Pray unceasingly for the world,
     quidem.
Unsoil the spirit. Rest when you fall down. Only then, take earth scent in,
     in moderation.

Free education should not be taken lightly. Especially when Physics has
     been chosen
over Hermeneutics. Nay! Your class of observation need not entail the
     fornication of mice!
Plants should display equally the discontinuity of atom, God's good
     benefaction.

II

And yet your work is incomplete and unconvincing. What's this, about the
   presence
of absences? The potential is there in the germ, the gene, you say, and
   evident
in only one of three grandchildren. The Good Lord Jesus was not a blend of
   his chaste parents?

Be that as it may, your research must be self-reflective—recessive. Perhaps
   it will resurface
in some generations, after you have assumed the role of Abbott. Indeed, yes
   paperwork,
as much as robes, could snag, but you have amply proven hardihood.

III

Genius, as it were, must be—like God—invisibly existent. Just
   unexpressed,
for now, until He recrudesces. Perhaps your lifework will revivify from the
   luckless bonfire,
unscathed; your papers, after all, did lie on Darwin's bookshelf when he
   died; alas, uncut.

References

23andMe (2014) 'An update for 23andMe customers', 31 March, available at
   http://blog.23andme.com/news/an-fda-update-for-23andme-customers (accessed 4
   August 2015).
23andMe (2015a) '23andMe therapeutics', 12 March, available at http://blog.23andme.com/
   news/23andme-therapeutics (accessed 4 August 2015).
23andMe (2015b) 'Learn how your DNA may affect your health', www.23andme.com/en-
   gb/health (accessed 18 September 2015).
Abbate, J. (2000) *Inventing the internet*, Cambridge, MA: MIT Press.
Adams, S. (2010) 'Sourcing the crowd for health experiences: Letting the people speak or
   obliging voice through choice?', in R. Harris, N. Wathen and S. Wyatt (eds),
   *Configuring health consumers: Health work and the imperative of personal responsi-
   bility*, Basingstoke: Palgrave Macmillan, pp. 178–193.
Agar, J. (2006) 'What difference did computers make to science?', *Social Studies of
   Science*, vol. 36, pp. 869–907.
Allison, M. (2009) 'Can web 2.0 reboot clinical trials?', *Nature Biotechnology*, vol. 27, no.
   10, pp. 895–902.
Arnquist, S. (2009) 'Research trove: Patients' online data', *New York Times*, 24 August,
   available at www.nytimes.com/2009/08/25/health/25web.html?pagewanted=all
   (accessed 2 September 2015).

Borgman, C. (2015) *Big data, little data, no data*, Cambridge, MA: MIT Press.

Borry, P. and Howard, H. (2008) 'DTC genetic services: A look across the pond', *American Journal of Bioethics*, vol. 8, no. 6, pp. 14–16, doi: 10.1080/15265160802248252.

Burrows, R., Nettleton, S., Pleace, N., Loader, B. and Muncer, B. (2000) 'Virtual community care: Social policy and the emergence of computer mediated social support', *Information, Communication and Society*, vol. 3, no. 1, pp. 95–121, doi: 10.1080/136911800359446.

Chial, H. (2008) 'Rare genetic disorders: Learning about genetic disease through gene mapping, SNPs, and microarray data', *Nature Education*, vol. 1, no. 1, p. 192.

Christensen, H. and Hickie, I. B. (2010) 'Using e-health applications to deliver new mental health services', *Medical Journal of Australia*, vol. 192, no. 11, pp. S53–S56.

Contreras, Jorge L. (2010) 'Bermuda's legacy: Policy, patents and the design of the genome commons', *Minnesota Journal of Law, Science and Technology*, vol. 12, p. 61.

Cox, S. M. and McKellin, W. (1999) '"There's this thing in our family": Predictive testing and the construction of risk for Huntington Disease', *Sociology of Health and Illness*, vol. 21, no. 5, pp. 622–646.

Davies, K. (2002) *Cracking the genome: Inside the race to unlock human DNA*, Baltimore, MD: Johns Hopkins University Press.

Dedding, C., van Doorn, R., Winkler, L. and Reis, R. (2011) 'How will e-health affect patient participation in the clinic? A review of e-health studies and the current evidence for changes in the relationship between medical professionals and patients', *Social Science and Medicine*, vol. 72, no. 1, pp. 49–53.

Dingel, M., Ostergen, J. McCormick, J., Hammer, R. and Koenig, B. (2015) 'The media and behavioral genetics: Alternatives coexisting with addiction genetics', *Science, Technology and Human Values*, vol. 40, no. 4, pp. 459–486.

Fearnley, L. (2006) 'Beyond the public's health: Constructing national syndromic surveillance', working paper, Anthropology of the Contemporary Research Collaboratory, available at http://citeseerx.ist.psu.edu/viewdoc/summary?doi=10.1.1.113.3472 (accessed 2 September 2015).

Fortun, M. (2008) *Promising Genomics: Iceland and DeCODE Genetics in a World of Speculation*, Berkeley, CA: University of California Press.

Foster, V. and Young, A. (2012) 'The use of routinely collected patient data for research: A critical review', *Health*, vol. 16, no. 4, pp. 448–463.

Frank, L. (2011) *My beautiful genome: Exposing our genetic future, one quirk at a time*, Oxford: Oneworld.

Gannett, L. (2014) 'The Human Genome Project', *Stanford Encyclopedia of Philosophy*, winter, Edward N. Zalta (ed.), available at http://plato.stanford.edu/archives/win2014/entries/human-genome (accessed 18 September 2015).

Ginsberg, J., Mohebbi, M. H., Patel, R. S., Brammer, L., Smolinski, M. S. and Brilliant, L. (2009) 'Detecting influenza epidemics using search engine query data', *Nature*, vol. 457, pp. 1012–1014.

Goetz, T. (2010) 'Sergey Brin's search for a Parkinson's cure', *Wired*, 6 December, available at www.wired.com/2010/06/ff_sergeys_search (accessed 19 September 2015).

Goldberg, G. (2011) 'Rethinking the public/virtual sphere: The problem with participation', *New Media and Society*, vol. 13, no. 5, pp. 739–754.

Guttmacher, A. E. and Collins, F. S. (2003) 'Welcome to the genomic era', *New England Journal of Medicine*, vol. 349, no. 10, pp. 996–998, doi: 10.1056/NEJMe038132.

Hardey, M. (1999) 'Doctor in the house: The Internet as a source of lay health knowledge and the challenge to expertise', *Sociology of Health and Illness*, vol. 21, no. 6, pp. 820–835, doi: 10.1111/1467-9566.00185.

Harper, M. (2015) 'Surprise! With $60 million Genentech deal, 23andMe has a business plan', *Forbes Business*, 6 January.

Hedgecoe, A. (2001) 'Schizophrenia and the narrative of enlightened geneticization', *Social Studies of Science*, vol. 31, no. 6, pp. 875–911.

Helmreich, S. (2009) *Alien ocean: Anthropological voyages in microbial seas*, Berkeley, CA: University of California Press.

Hine, C. (2006) 'Databases as scientific instruments and their role in the ordering of scientific work', *Social Studies of Science*, vol. 36, no. 2, pp. 269–298.

Hunter, D. J., Khoury, M. J. and Drazen, J. M. (2008) 'Letting the genome out of the bottle – will we get our wish?', *New England Journal of Medicine*, vol. 358, no. 2, pp. 105–107.

Ihde, D. (2002) *Bodies in technologies*, Minneapolis, MN: University of Minnesota Press.

Jenkins, H. (2006) *Convergence culture: Where old and new media collide*, New York, NY: New York University Press.

Kaplan, K., Salzer, M. S., Solomon, P., Brusilovskiy, E. and Cousounis, P. (2011) 'Internet peer support for individuals with psychiatric disabilities: A randomized controlled trial', *Social Science and Medicine*, vol. 72, no. 1, pp. 54–62.

Kerr, A. and Shakespeare, T. (2002) *Genetic politics: From eugenics to genome*, Cheltenham: New Clarion Press.

Kevles, D. and Hood, L. (1993) *The code of codes: Scientific and social issues in the Human Genome Project.* Cambridge, MA: Harvard University Press.

Kitchin, R. (2014) *The data revolution: Big data, open data, data infrastructures and their consequences*, New York: Sage.

König, R. (2013) 'Wikipedia: Between lay participation and elite knowledge representation', *Information Communication and Society*, vol. 16, no. 2, pp. 160–177.

Kroes, N. (2014) 'Video: EU-commissioner Neelie Kroes on mHealth', available at https://ec.europa.eu/digital-agenda/en/news/video-commissioner-neelie-kroes-mhealth (accessed 14 April 2015).

Lee, S. S. (2013) 'American DNA: The politics of potentiality in a genomic age', *Current Anthropology*, vol. 54, supplement 7, pp. S77–S86.

Lee, S. S., Vernez, S. L., Ormond, K. E. and Granovetter, M. (2013) 'Attitudes towards social networking and sharing behaviors among consumers of direct-to-consumer personal genomics', *Journal of Personalized Medicine*, vol. 3, no. 4, pp. 275–287.

Lemire, M., Sicotte, C. and Paré, G. (2008) 'Internet use and the logics of personal empowerment in health', *Health Policy*, vol. 88, no. 1, pp. 130–140.

Leonelli, S. (2012) 'When humans are the exception: cross-species databases at the interface of biological and clinical research', *Social Studies of Science*, vol. 42, no. 2, pp. 214–236.

Lippman, A. (1991) 'Prenatal genetic testing and screening: Constructing needs and reinforcing inequalities', *American Journal of Law and Medicine*, vol. 17, nos 1–2, pp. 15–50.

Lock, M., Freeman, J., Sharples, R. and Lloyd, S. (2006) 'When it runs in the family: Putting susceptibility genes in perspective', *Public Understanding of Science*, vol. 15, no. 3, pp. 277–300.

Lupton, D. (2012) 'The quantified self movement: some sociological perspectives', *This Sociological Life: A blog by sociologist Deborah Lupton*, available at https://simplysociology.wordpress.com/2012/11/04/the-quantitative-self-movement-some-sociological -perspectives (accessed 19 September 2015]

McGowan, M. L., Fishman, J. R. and Lambrix, M. A. (2010) 'Personal genomics and individual identities: Motivations and moral imperatives of early users', *New Genetics and Society*, vol. 29, no. 3, pp. 261–290, doi: 10.1080/14636778.2010.507485.

McGuire, A. L., Diaz, C. M., Wang, T. and Hilsenbeck, S. G. (2009) 'Social networkers' attitudes toward direct-to-consumer personal genome testing', *The American Journal of Bioethics*, vol. 9, nos 6–7, pp. 3–10.

Martin, E. (2007) *Bipolar expeditions: Mania and depression in American culture*, Princeton, NJ: Princeton University Press.

Meropol, N. J., Daly, M., Vig, H., Manion, F., Manne, S., Mazar, C., Murphy, C., Solarino, N. and Zubarev, V. (2011) 'Delivery of internet-based cancer genetic counselling services to patients' homes: A feasibility study', *Journal of Telemedicine and Telecare*, vol. 17, no. 1, pp. 36–40.

Mort, M., May, C. R. and Williams, T. (2003) 'Remote doctors and absent patients: Acting at a distance in telemedicine?', *Science, Technology and Human Values*, vol. 28, no. 2, pp. 274–295.

Munro, D. (2013) 'Class action lawsuit filed against 23andMe', *Forbes Business*, 3 December, available at www.forbes.com/sites/danmunro/2013/12/02/class-action-lawsuit-filed-against-23andme (accessed 24 April 2015).

Nature (2001) 'What a long strange trip it's been ...', *Nature*, vol. 409, 15 February, pp. 756–757, doi:10.1038/35057286.

Niederer, S. and van Dijck, J. (2010) 'Wisdom of the crowd or technicity of content? Wikipedia as a sociotechnical system', *New Media and Society*, vol. 12, no. 8, pp. 1368–1387.

Nowotny, H., Scott, P. and Gibbons, M. (2001) *Re-thinking science: Knowledge and the public in an age of uncertainty*, Cambridge, UK: Polity.

O'Reilly, T. (2005) 'What is web 2.0? Design patterns and business models for the next generation of software', available at http://oreilly.com/web2/archive/what-is-web-20.html (accessed 12 August 2015).

O'Riordan, K. (2013) 'Biodigital publics: Personal genomes as digital media artifacts', *Science as Culture*, vol. 22, no. 4, pp. 516–539.

Oudshoorn, N. (2008) 'Diagnosis at a distance: The invisible work of patients and health-care professionals in cardiac telemonitoring technology', *Sociology of Health and Illness*, vol. 30, no. 2, pp. 272–288.

Oudshoorn, N. (2011) *Telecare technologies and the transformation of healthcare*, Basingstoke: Palgrave Macmillan.

Oudshoorn, N. (2012) 'How places matter: Telecare technologies and the changing spatial dimensions of healthcare', *Social Studies of Science*, vol. 42, no. 1, pp. 121–142.

Pálsson, G. (2009) 'Biosocial relations of production', *Comparative Studies in Society and History*, vol. 51, no. 2, pp. 288–313.

Paul, D. B. (1998) 'Genetic screening, economics, and eugenics', *Science in Context*, vol. 11, pp. 93–99.

Pels, D. (2003) *Unhastening science: Autonomy and reflexivity in the social theory of knowledge*, Liverpool: University of Liverpool Press.

Peterson, A. and Lupton, D. (1996) *The new public health: Discourse, knowledges and strategies*, London: Sage.

Pols, J. (2011) 'Wonderful webcams: About active gazes and invisible technologies', *Science, Technology and Human Values*, vol. 36, no. 4, pp. 451–473.

Prainsack, B. (2011) 'Voting with their mice: Personal genome testing and the "participatory turn" in disease research', *Accountability in Research*, vol. 18, no. 3, pp. 132–147.

Proulx, S., Heaton, L., Kwok Choon, M. J. and Millette, M. (2011) 'Paradoxical empowerment of *produsers* in the context of informational capitalism', *New Review of Hypermedia and Multimedia*, vol. 17, no. 1, pp. 9–29.

Savage, M. and Burrows, R. (2007) 'The coming crisis of empirical sociology', *Sociology*, vol. 41, no. 5, pp. 885-899.

Shifman, L. (2012) 'An anatomy of a YouTube meme', *New Media and Society*, vol. 14, no. 2, pp. 187–203.

Singer, E. (2007) 'Your personal genome: George Church wants to sequence your genome', *MIT Technology Review*, 6 December, available at www.technologyreview.com/news/409153/your-personal-genome (accessed 24 April 2015).

Smithsonian (no date) 'Timeline of the human genome', Smithsonian National Museum of Natural History in partnership with National Human Genome Research Institute, available at http://unlockinglifescode.org/timeline?tid=4 (accessed 4 August 2015).

Surowiecki, J. (2004) *The wisdom of crowds: Why the many are smarter than the few and how collective wisdom shapes business, economies, societies and nations*, London: Little, Brown.

Swan, M., Hathaway, K. Hogg, C., MacCaulay, R., and Vollrath, A. (2010) 'Citizen science genomics as a model for crowdsourced preventive medicine research', *Journal of Participatory Medicine*, vol. 2, 23 December, available at www.jopm.org/evidence/research/2010/12/23/citizen-science-genomics-as-a-model-for-crowdsourced-preventive-medicine-research (accessed September 20 2015).

Tapscott, D. and Williams, A. (2006) *Wikinomics: How mass collaboration changes everything*, New York: Portfolio.

Telegraph (2009) 'DNA father James Watson's "holy grail" request', 10 May, available at www.telegraph.co.uk/news/worldnews/northamerica/usa/5300883/DNA-father-James-Watsons-holy-grail-request.html (accessed 18 September 2015).

Terranova, T. (2000) 'Free labor: Producing culture for the digital economy', *Social Text*, vol. 18, no. 2, pp. 33–58.

Thomas, G. and Wyatt, S. (1999) 'Shaping cyberspace: Interpreting and transforming the internet', *Research Policy*, vol. 28, pp. 681–698.

Tutton, R. (2014) *Genomics and the reimagining of personalized medicine*, London: Ashgate.

US Federal Trade Commission (2006) 'Direct to consumer genetic tests', available at www.consumer.ftc.gov/articles/0166-direct-consumer-genetic-tests (accessed 24 April 2015).

Veatch, P. M., LeRoy, B. S. and Bartels, D. M. (2003) *Facilitating the practice of genetic counseling: A practice manual*, New York, NY: Springer.

Wathen, N., Wyatt, S. and Harris, R. (eds) (2008) *Mediating health information: The go-betweens in a changing socio-technical landscape*, Basingstoke: Palgrave Macmillan.

Wesch, M. (2008) 'An anthropological introduction to YouTube', available AT www.youtube.com/watch?v=TPAO-lZ4_hU (accessed 4 August 2015).

Wicks, P., Vaughan, T. E., Massagli, M. P. and Heywood, J. (2011) 'Accelerated clinical discovery using self-reported patient data collected online and a patient-matching algorithm', *Nature Biotechnology*, vol. 29, no. 5, pp. 411–414.

Wiener, N. (1948/1961) *Cybernetics or control and communication in the animal and the machine*, 2nd edition, Cambridge, MA: MIT Press.

Woolgar, S. (2002) 'Five rules of virtuality', in S. Woolgar (ed.), *Virtual society? Technology, cyberpole, reality*, Oxford: Oxford University Press, pp. 1–22.

Wouters, P., Beaulieu, A., Scharnhorst, A. and Wyatt, S. (eds) (2013) *Virtual knowledge:*

Experimenting in the humanities and the social sciences, Cambridge, MA: The MIT Press.

Wyatt, S. (2008) 'Technological determinism is dead; long live technological determinism', in E. Hackett, O. Amsterdamska, M. Lynch and J. Wajcman (eds), *Handbook of Science and Technology Studies*, Cambridge, MA: MIT Press, pp. 165–180.

Wyatt, S., Harris, A. and Kelly, S. (2016) 'Controversy goes online: Schizophrenia genetics on Wikipedia', *Science and Technology Studies*, vol. 2, no. 1, pp. 13-29.

Wyatt, S., Thomas, G. and Terranova, T. (2002) 'They came, they surfed, they went back to the beach: Conceptualising use and non-use of the Internet', in S. Woolgar (ed.), *Virtual society? Technology, cyberbole, reality*, Oxford: Oxford University Press, pp. 23–40.

2   Users

In order to understand more about the socio-temporal relations being configured and reconfigured with online genetic testing, we turn first to the users of these services. As scholars in the field of STS have highlighted, users are integral to the co-construction of technologies in everyday life; that is, users matter (Oudshoorn and Pinch, 2005a). Users not only consume technologies but also modify, domesticate, design and resist technologies. This becomes evident in practices, not only practices of use but also those of non-use (Wyatt, 2005). We will find evidence of such practices in this chapter, looking at how individuals engage in scripted and creative ways with online genetic testing. Technologies also shape users. Again, in this book we examine the ways in which markets, companies, the internet, skills and other technological arrangements shape users of online genetic testing. The co-construction of users and technologies highlights the limitations of deterministic discourses on technologies and essentialist perspectives about users (Oudshoorn and Pinch, 2005b).

Who becomes defined as a user and who makes this definition? In this book various kinds of actors will appear who are defined as users by companies, in their own accounts and in the academic literature (including our own research, see more in Appendix A):

- individuals who order the tests;
- genetic counsellors and physicians who use online genetic testing either through their employment or engagement with patients and clients;
- advertisers;
- curious researchers;
- the genetic testing companies (as users themselves of services); and
- potential users (people living with a diagnosis of a mental disorder), among others.

These users are described in different ways, which is highly revealing about how they are conceptualised by the different actors involved. For example, a user who buys the tests might be described as a 'consumer', highlighting the commercial nature of the activities individuals are engaging in when they go online. National contexts become important – while individuals in the US have for some time been considered consumers of healthcare, this takes shape differently in different places of the world. It is becoming increasingly common however, for users of healthcare services globally to become consumers of technologies. Part of their role as consumers means users paying for a service, such as to have their genetic results analysed from a sample of spit that they provide. This relationship of consumer-provider becomes blurred however once we dig further into our analysis of online genetic testing; for example as users start providing further data to the company through engaging in their research paradigms. In this context, the user is reconfigured as research subject, as they become one of many in aggregated data sets used for research purposes. This dual role comes with its own complexities, especially considering the ways in which such involvement in research is branded by the companies as 'participatory' and a form of citizen engagement. We explore these complexities in greater detail in Chapter 4.

While much could be said about the range of different actors described as users in online genetic testing, and we explore some of these further in the next chapter on healthcare providers, in this chapter we focus on users as individuals who have paid to have genetic testing through an internet-based company. Something that became very clear in our own analysis of DTC genetic testing websites is that these users were not clearly defined as 'patients'. Or rather, their engagement in the online genetic testing process was not framed in regards to being a patient. First the companies did not want to frame their users in this way, for it risked bringing the company under regulation from national authorities for providing a medical test. As we have seen in the opening chapter of this book, this has caused difficulties for one company in particular, that was ordered to stop selling their tests because of the health claims made on the websites. Second, as we found in our empirical research, users of genetic tests online did not frame themselves as patients either. As we explore through the example of videos uploaded by users of 23andMe later in this chapter, many aspects of patienthood were not found in their narratives. The users were not unwell or suffering. They were curious and rarely connect to specific disease categories or conditions.

This absence of connection with medical conditions and the limited connection with others with the same medical conditions causes us to question whether we are indeed witnessing here the form of biosociality that many have predicted and observed in relation to technologies such as online genetic testing (Rose and Novas, 2005). Biosociality was initially considered by Rabinow (1996) as the possible arrangement of groups formed around life at the molecular level, through chromosomes and alleles, where those with shared genetics would develop shared traditions and narratives to help understand their fate. The term was further developed by Rose and Novas (2005) to tend more to the identity politics entangled with technological transformations in healthcare, focusing particularly on the movement from patient to active citizen, through subscribing to and utilising medical categories. There have been a number of critiques of the term biosociality including its over-emphasis on newness, and the reduction of complex social processes to biology (Kerr, 2004; Plows and Boddington, 2006; Raman and Tutton, 2010). While we do not have room here to tease apart the evolution of the term biosociality or its critiques, we suggest a new term as an alternative way of considering the stories told around engagements with new healthcare technologies: autobiology.

'Autobiology' is the term we use to describe the study of and story about one's own organism. Derived from the term autobiography, this is a story that encompasses the biological; a study of one's life including the molecular, the cellular, the genetic, the physiological and/or other biological elements. We argue that such autobiologies are told in the context of encounters with one's own biology that are being reconfigured with the introduction of new technologies.

There are several features of autobiology. First, they are stories about technologies where testing and monitoring of healthcare has to some extent travelled outside the clinic. Second, the context of storytelling differs from the more classical sociological genre of the illness narrative, in that the storytellers are not framed principally as patients, as they are not unwell. Third, autobiologies are characterised by a temporal engagement with health, illness and biology. Again, unlike pathobiographies or illness narratives where illness becomes an important part of one's identity, autobiologies are fleeting engagements. Fourth, unlike the narratives of patient activist groups, who use stories as a powerful means for influencing community research and therapeutic agendas, autobiologies focus very much on the individual, on the self. As such, there are elements of narcissism and performance of celebrity or micro-celebrity (Marwick and boyd, 2011a, 2011b). Stories may be connected, but not through a shared patient experience or diagnosis but rather through shared engagements with technological platforms, a form of collective individualism occurring in the context of networked publics (boyd, 2014).

In this chapter we use the term autobiology to further tease out the ways in which users are being configured by and configuring online genetic testing. We position our discussion within a growing body of literature that examines not patients but new kinds of 'patients in waiting' (Timmermans and Buchbinder, 2010), the emerging states of hovering between sickness and health, states characterised by the uncertainties entangled with many medical technologies. We examine this liminal state by looking at the stories told by users of genetic testing services. Stories are useful ways in which to examine how users define themselves and their technological practices.

In this chapter, autobiology helps to capture narratives told at the molecular level, stories which concern genetic markers, alleles and ribonucleic acids, interweaving family histories of illness into wayfaring (Ingold, 2007) narratives. They are also autobiological narratives in the ways in which they document a sense of self-making through forms of biological practice and scientific experimentation entailed in the genetic testing process, practices which exhibit a form of playfulness, while simultaneously being bound up with consumerist concerns. We will examine these issues through two kinds of user accounts: the first, that of a celebrity genetic testing user, the Danish journalist Lone Frank, who wrote about her experiences of undergoing online genetic testing in an autobiography. There are a number of celebrity accounts of undergoing genetic testing in novels and magazine articles (see also Pinker, 2009) but these are now becoming vastly outnumbered by stories from users with different kinds of public profiles, who may not be nationally or internationally renowned because of their jobs but rather develop their presence online in other ways. We call this group the 'non-celebrity' users. In the second part of the chapter we examine these non-celebrity users who posted their stories of online genetic testing online, on the internet platform YouTube.

In delineating between the celebrity user account in a book form and non-celebrity users documenting their stories on YouTube, we remain aware that the ways in which celebrities are constructed in contemporary society is dynamic and performative. Increased access to technologies including the internet has led to techniques of 'micro-celebrity' (Marwick and boyd 2011a) for example, which entails using social media to maintain audiences. Celebrity and non-celebrity cannot be clearly distinguished but rather seen as a set of performed practices (Marwick and boyd, 2011b). Nonetheless, in order to help with our analysis of two different bodies of research material we make the categorisation in this chapter of 'celebrity' as widely famous individuals and 'non-celebrity' as individuals who are not in the global media spotlight. The storytelling genre that emerges however is very similar in both accounts, demonstrating potentially new ways in which users are engaging with healthcare technologies both as celebrities, including micro-celebrities, and regular users. In the accounts of online genetic testing we discuss in this chapter, the context of storytelling differs from the more classical sociological genre of the illness narrative, in that the storytellers were not framed principally as patients; as we introduced at the beginning of the chapter, they differed from patients in that they were not unwell. In order to better situate these narratives, we turn to a body of literature which examines a liminal state entangled with emerging healthcare technologies such as online genetic testing, where concepts such as 'partial patients', 'proto-disease' and 'patients-in-waiting' have been introduced.

Patients-in-waiting

'Partial patients' refers to people who do not feel ill, most or all of the time, but who have been informed that because of certain characteristics they may have a disease, or be at risk of getting the disease (Greaves, 2000). 'Proto-disease' has been described in reference to asymptomatic conditions such as hypertension and hypercholesterolemia (Rosenberg, 2009). Timmermans and Buchbinder (2010) use the umbrella term 'patients-in-waiting' to capture both of these concepts, as well as individuals on a spectrum of disease, such as autism. In a similar vein, Novas and Rose (2000) have discussed the 'genetically at risk'. These are all emerging states between risk factor and manifest illness, a hovering between sickness and health characterised by uncertainty. Timmermans and Buchbinder (2010) argue that 'in-waiting' will be a persistent form of liminality in contemporary healthcare, one that can be seen to have emerged with technologies of medical surveillance (Adams, 2013; Armstrong, 1995). While their description of patients-in-waiting being on 'a rollercoaster ride between alarm and hope' (Timmermans and Buchbinder, 2010: 418), at the mercy of health policies and medical gatekeeping, does not apply directly to users engaging with genetic testing (for, as will become apparent, they were very casual about their results) the kinds of narratives we discuss in this chapter could be broadly categorised into these emerging states of illness liminality.

The convergence of the internet and genetics in DTC genetic testing that we explore throughout this book means that it is pertinent to consider the digital nature of storytelling about these issues. The autobiologies we examined on YouTube are digital narratives, told, uploaded, shared and discussed through the internet, via webcams (Miller and Sinanan, 2013) and other devices. The internet and related technologies allow for new kinds of self-expression, through the use of written and spoken words, images (moving or still), hyperlinks, avatars and other online features. At the time of writing this book the study of digital illness narratives is still in its infancy. Researchers who have examined how individuals are engaging with YouTube for health and illness issues have looked at, for example, obesity (Yoo and Kim, 2011), organ donation (Tian, 2010) cancer survivorship (Chou *et al.*, 2011) and anorexia (Syed-Abdul *et al.*, 2013). Rather than examine narratives however, these studies focus on the role of these videos in health promotion and raising public awareness, how they provide information and support, and potentially change behaviour. Further qualitative research has been conducted on the video narratives posted on the HealthTalkOnline website (Newman, Ziebland and Barker, 2009). These are interviews about particular health conditions, videos made by researchers or videographers. We are interested in individuals' self-made narratives about the experience of genetic testing. Our work relates closely to O'Riordan's work on biodigital lives, emerging from 'a new field of biographical and autobiographical tales *from* the genome' (2011: 127) which is crossing multiple media forms.

In this chapter we build upon and contribute new insights to a body of literature about digital narratives and patients-in-waiting by drawing on our own empirical study of narratives about DTC genetic testing. In *The Wounded Storyteller*, Arthur Frank (1995) writes that there are more narratives to be found about illness than the three that he identifies and which are most commonly drawn upon by social scientists in illness narrative analysis. We take Arthur Frank up on this provocation and consider what other kinds of stories of and by users there are to be found in relation to genetic testing. We consider these accounts of users in regards to the content of the stories, the way they are being told, and the circumstances of the telling, including their performativity. We do not claim to 'capture' context in doing so, but rather provide insights into aspects of users' practices, whether that be the celebrity users or non-celebrity users on YouTube.

Celebrity users

During New York Fashion Week 2008, 23andMe hosted the world's first 'spit party'. *Mother Jones* magazine dubbed the glamorous salivaters who attended this event the 'spitterati' (Darnovsky, 2008). With cocktail glasses teetering in one hand and a spittoon in the other, the smartly dressed crowd leaned over somewhat awkwardly in their tight dresses and jackets to spit. These users were some of the early adopters of DTC genetic testing, part of the high-tech world of latest gadgets, with privileged access to new technologies in hope that their trendsetting may lead to broader diffusion. In trying to learn more about the users of online genetic testing, we began by looking at the accounts of these celebrity users. There have been a number who have documented their genetic testing experiences and the one we focus on here is the Danish science journalist Lone Frank (2011a), specifically her book *My Beautiful Genome: Exposing our Genetic Future, One Quirk at a Time* (previously published in Danish as *Mit Smukke Genome*).

In *My Beautiful Genome*, Lone Frank documents her search for information about her genetic past, present, and future. The underlying message of her book is that genes are not our destiny but something we can 'work with', something Frank examines through her search for traces of genetic associations that explain her own family history of depression. Lone Frank's father often told her that while she had many 'trophies on the shelves' (2011a: 6) in the genetics department, she did inherit some 'bad' genes from both her parents in regards to depression. Describing herself as an 'incurable melancholic' (2011a: 207), Frank details an 'unbroken line' of depression in her family. Her great-grandfather killed himself, his daughter (her grandmother) almost had a lobotomy, her mother suffered from depression, her father was 'manic-depressive' and attempted suicide twice, and her brother has depression too. Counting both sides, Frank declares, her family boasts three successful suicides. In the book, Frank focuses doggedly on the many avenues available to her to find out about her own genetic predisposition to depression and other traits and illnesses.

The lengths Frank goes to in this search are impressive. She undertakes genome sequencing and personality tests for a Copenhagen University Hospital research project examining the connection between specific genes and depression. She is tested by Icelandic genetic testing company deCODEme and mines her raw data for genetic associations found in the scientific literature. She has blood tests in order to take part in research by a pharmaceutical company looking for biomarkers for mental illness. Along the way Frank also undertakes several other activities:

- she signs up for a free 23andMe account;
- she takes an ancestry test offered by an American firm wanting to recruit Scandinavians;
- she has a genetic test for breast cancer (which requires pestering and convincing the clinical geneticist to run a full BRCA sequence); and
- she finally takes a test for genetic romantic compatibility.

Frank pulls others, including her brother, into being tested to aid her genetic search, while she is pulled into the romantic matching test by a work colleague, having her (Frank's) boyfriend tested at the same time.

The comparative findings of these tests are interesting, for they provide very different, and sometimes contrasting, pictures of Lone Frank's psychiatric genetic makeup. Mining her deCODEme raw data reveals an increased risk of depression, while the personality test tells her that according to her neuroticism score she is 'not particularly inclined towards depression' (2011a: 206). Later on her blood biomarkers put her 'solidly in the group of depressed research subjects', while the genetic analysis run by the Copenhagen University Hospital tells her that she has two short variants of the SERT gene (responsible for serotonin transportation), findings which show a particular vulnerability to depression in association with 'unfortunate life circumstances' (2011a: 219). The test also shows that she has a double dose of the 'worrier' variant of the COMT gene, variants of the BDNF gene which make her sensitive to stress and two copies of a less efficient MAOA variant which predisposes women to depression. The university research results seem to be the most reliable findings for Frank – she throws her pen on the table when hearing the news: 'So my damned recurring depressions don't just come from nowhere' (2011a: 219). She recognises the uncertainty of these findings but nonetheless considers herself a 'pitiful loser in the genetic lottery' (2011a: 223).

In her account, Frank not only discusses the results but what it is like to go through the genetic testing process. She describes what fun it was to receive the deCODEme swabbing material in the mail, scrape her cheek and send the sample back to Reykjavik for analysis. The fun dissipates when she receives her results, in a hotel room, alone. Frank opens a can of beer for company. She feels certain that the test is going to report a high risk of breast cancer and keeps her eyes closed, long after she has clicked on the results. Finding out that she has a lower than average risk, she engages in descriptive determinism as she feels 'as if a very old, hissing pressure deep inside [her] body quickly seeps out and floats away' (2011a: 77). She pores over the rest of her results, well into the long Icelandic night, later digging into her raw data over a series of late evenings on sites like Promethease. The uncertainty, fear and waiting involved in genetic testing is captured well when Frank describes waiting for her breast cancer gene sequencing results and experiencing diarrhoea all weekend.

*My Beautiful Geno*me is personal, but mostly at the molecular level. Frank's story is *biological*. When she talks about her interest in the human being as an organism, she does not refer here to an individual living in a rich social environment as an anthropologist or geographer might, but rather to the 'microscopic processes unfolding' within us (2011a: 5). Even the 'godfather of genetics', James Watson, admits in an interview with Frank that genetics are not central to his understanding of self. In response to her question about how knowing his genome has affected him, he replies 'to be honest, I don't think much about it' (2011a: 17). Lone Frank is on a quest, which could be seen as a search not only for genetic truth, but also to understand herself through new technologies and gadgets, whether they are related to genetics or to neuroscience. This quest though is different from the kinds of quest narratives we find from patients. In the book Lone Frank makes sense of her life and her lineage through biology her story told from a 'molecular gaze' (Rose, 2007) centring around ribonucleic acid and the array of technologies tied up with understanding the body at this level. This way of describing one's use of genetic testing services, what we term autobiology, is not unique to this celebrity. We also found autobiologies when we started looking into the stories and accounts of a now growing body of non-celebrity users of DTC genetic testing.

Non-celebrity users

The increasing number of users of genetic testing services across the world are documenting their stories not so often in books and magazine articles like the celebrities, but rather across a range of web-based media platforms available to them. Other researchers have examined individual testimonies about DTC genetic testing on blogs and on company websites (Nordgren and Juengst, 2009; Su, Howard and Borry, 2011). In our own research, we focused on YouTube videos posted by users of DTC genetic testing services in order to understand more about how people are engaging with this technology. YouTube provides access to users' stories in the public domain, with details about the process of undergoing testing and interpreting results, results which are their own rather than the hypothetical scenarios. It is a website, just like the genetic testing websites, where the individual meets the collective, where individual stories/genetic data are shared and discussed and the private is rendered public. Considering a collection of narratives about testing 'me', as in 23andMe, as autobiologies captured in, and on a 'you' tube, thus seemed particularly apt. As McGowan, Fishman and Lambrix (2010: 276) point out in their study of early adopters of genetic testing, it is important to consider how users of DTC genetic testing not only use the internet as a tool to purchase the product but also to comment on it.

The YouTube videos we analysed shared a range of features, some shared with YouTube videos more broadly such as amateur videography and focus on an 'ordinary person' (Shifman, 2012). Irrespective of whether the videos were filmed with a stationary webcam or by someone with a handheld camera, they mostly focused on one person, except for one video of a spit party in which multiple users were visible. This collection of videos was posted by 17 predominantly young North Americans. We met PandyFackleresque, or Pandy for short. Pandy had a new Mohawk haircut, multiple piercings, tattoos and posted one 'spitting' video and one 'logging in' video. Another YouTuber who has posted two videos was Jen McCabe, a health 2.0 activist championing the 23andMe Research Revolution. There was also Zyloga, a psychology major who provided a more cynical critique of the company's activities; and Eric, who was somewhat surprised when he received his spit kit in the mail as a gift from friends. The videos were set in bedrooms, home studies, workplaces, a dining room, a university common room and a sun deck, all places becoming in some ways at-home biological 'laboratories'. In the bedrooms it was possible to see messy, unmade beds, posters on the walls and wine bottles. A cat climbed the stairs in the background of one video and ran back down. Other backgrounds were littered with computer hardware.

All videos were edited on a number of levels. The footage itself was edited, mostly concerning the 'spitting' moments either being deleted or 'sped up'. The videos were also edited regarding which aspects of the genetic results the individuals chose to share, attempts at maintaining privacy by covering up names or birth dates, and other editing of storylines. Some videos were enhanced with soundtracks and hyperlinks (to 23andMe, blogs, Wikipedia pages and Twitter accounts). As well as linking across internet platforms, the videos were interlaced with technological hardware such as other computers and printers. The computers may have been visible in the background, a computer screen the focus of the video, or the camera capturing the view from the computer, the presence of the screen just a blue glow on someone's face. Other technologies make an appearance such as iPhones and iPods – Zyloga has uploaded her genetic results onto her iPod so that she can carry it around with her, while Florian times his spitting on his iPhone (it takes eight minutes), taking a call mid-way through the video: 'Hey Tracey, what's up? [pause] I am spitting into a cup.' The YouTubers were constantly moving between a range of other texts: the 23andMe website text (read out, scrolled through, hyperlinks clicked) and the leaflet that arrives with the spit kit explaining how to collect the saliva sample. They also used a number of objects, such as 23andMe boxes and the spittoon, objects which featured most prominently in videos which we explore in more detail in the following section.

'This is pretty disgusting but I would like to share it with you': sense-making through biological practices

Jen was sitting at her office desk in a bright pink t-shirt, city lights sparkling beyond a large window behind her, also reflecting someone holding a video camera. She was filmed excitedly rubbing her cheeks and spitting into a tube. In his home study Eric opened a FedEx box. He continued to glance simultaneously at a YouTube music video on his computer screen (a YouTube within a YouTube), 'The Final Countdown' building cinematic climax as he reached to find the spit kit (a tube within a box). Nick was also opening a box, laying out its contents on a table in neat parallel and perpendicular lines, then registering his details on a computer framed by a haphazard assemblage of Post-It notes. In a busy common room a group of university students were having a spit contest to see who could fill the 'crazy looking tubes' the fastest. Florian described what everyone was doing:

> I received this [spittoon] from 23andMe. This is the thing you have to spit in. You are not allowed to smoke, chew gum or eat 30 minutes before putting your saliva in this thing. This thing here [spittoon lid] is filled with liquid, so don't close that, as soon as you close it the liquid goes in the tube [reads out from instructions, gets comfortable on the chair] Relax, and rub your cheeks gently for 30 seconds to create saliva. [Rubs his cheeks with his hands. Leans forward to spit, video skips to him showing the tube half full.] … OK next step, spit, until the amount of saliva, not bubbles … close the lid, snap, unscrew the tube from the roof … pretty full huh, so don't fill too much

above the line. Pick up the small cap, and screw it on. Close tightly huh. Now shake for five seconds. Discard or recycle the blue funnel. We will discard. Put the sample tube in a plastic bag … There you go, it is closed, now this bag you put in this envelope which comes in your package, the rest you need is this [holds up form], and three copies of this [holds up another form], you put in this see-through thing and send.

Florian and many of the other YouTubers were filming themselves doing the work of DTC genetic testing. For many it was 'disgusting'. 'Oh that's gross, I don't like spit', Pandy exclaimed, then later, laughing, 'this is probably the grossest video I have ever made'. Some, like Florian, felt uncomfortable spitting on camera, others continually showing the spittoon as it 'filled up'. Many of them went about the process of testing diligently. They read the written instructions and rubbed their cheeks. Seen as a collection of videos the cheek rubbing and massaging almost became a form of ritualistic behaviour (Pace, 2008), as did 'unboxing' the package, all of these practices integrated into the testing experience. The YouTubers often took great care in filling up the tubes appropriately, sealing bags properly, finding barcodes and registering online. And like any 'good' patient about to have a clinical test, most made sure not to eat or drink half an hour before spitting. They posted the package, despite grumbles about FedEx; as Zyloga said, 'I'm mailing my spit to California'.

There was a script to these activities, in the sense of what was inscribed in the technology (Akrich, 1992), and also in regards to the spoken narrative about testing, in the form of a set of written instructions read out loud, sometimes twice, and constantly referred to. Like all scripts however, these instructions were not followed 'to the letter'. Instead, more mundane off-script events occurred, such as spilling the mixing solution in distracted moments, eating M&Ms before the test (turning one university student's saliva green), collecting spit in New York (but posting it from Massachusetts) and not always rubbing cheeks for 30 seconds. These kinds of scripted and non-scripted practices involved in creating a saliva sample for genetic analysis can be described as performing forms of biological practice, practices that are pseudo-clinical, in how the individual performs patient-like tasks, and also scientific, in their involvement in sample collection. The videos documented and provided tutorials about how to undertake these practices, offering 'handy hints' on ways to fill the tube, in the same way a YouTube tutorial on knitting may recommend stitch techniques. The videos gave context to the setting of these practices in a number of ways. They concerned the bodily nature of taking part in DTC genetic testing; the saliva created and users' embodied engagement with their computers for example. The context of these narratives also concerned the materiality of practices in regards to objects – boxes, tubes, the other vibrant matter (Bennett, 2010) of DTC genetic testing – and places in which these practices occur.

'Oh boy,' Jen exclaimed, 'you can see the solution mixing with the spit, very cool – it is like those oil and coloured water experiments in elementary and middle school science, very cool.' There was an air of experimentation being performed here. The experimental nature of DTC genetic testing was also evident in the *Nature* survey (Maher, 2011: 5), where 13.6 per cent of respondents reported to have engaged in forms of self-experimentation such as growing their own cells. In the case of the YouTube videos, the personal experience of undergoing genetic testing turned into a shared video experiment, the testing itself also experimental not only in relation to the symbolic association with test tubes, but also in regards to playing with a new technology. Videos had a backyard biopunk (Wohlsen, 2011) feel, the YouTubers referring to themselves as 'nerds' and 'geeks', amateur scientists revelling in the experimental nature of taking part in testing. Florian had posters of scientists such as Richard Feynman and Albert Einstein pinned up on his walls which he pointed out to the viewer. The biohazard bag for the spittoon becomes part of the experiment – 'I love this biohazard icon – oh man – to think that my spit is a biohazard!' Another said 'My favourite part about this sample bag is right there – biohazard – because my saliva is so dangerous – it makes me feel pretty cool, like I am in a post-apocalyptic world.' This YouTuber also commented bemusedly that he was surprised at how small the packaging of the spit kit was, and stated that he was half expecting a small laboratory to be delivered in the mail. These users all express forms of self-making through biology. We now examine other ways in which genetic testing users wove biology into their life stories.

'This is a home movie for the grandchildren to watch': wayfaring genetic narratives

Several months after uploading her unboxing/spitting video, Pandy uploaded a ten-minute video in which she shares her results. These two genetic testing videos were part of a collection of over 200 videos which she had uploaded about a range of topics, many of them science-related. At the time of our analysis, the video in which Pandy shared her genetic testing results had been viewed over 4,500 times. The video began with Pandy on her sun deck, logging into her account one week after she had received them. She gave a commentary of her results:

> The other things I have are chronic – ahh – lymphocytic leukaemia – not cool – high blood pressure, hypertension. That runs in my family so I kinda saw that one coming. However when I click on it to see exactly what they are talking about … [clicks on a hyperlink, reads out some web text, moves camera to the screen.] They even tell you where they found this on your genotype – I have to keep covering up my name here. These are the genes that they are talking about – GT, they found it on that specific one [camera reflected on screen, points to screen with her finger] … You can even go to which exact allele they are on … [increased glare on the screen] And of course it just got really sunny out. My decreased risks are type 2 diabetes, which is surprising since my maternal grandmother has that. But my risk is a 13.3 per cent, the average risk is 18.2 per cent so while it is a decreased risk, it is still not something that I don't need to look out for, especially since

it runs in the family. I also have a decreased risk of heart attack, psoriasis, melanoma, which is surprising because my father has melanoma. All kinds of stuff. They also list typical risks – so my risk for obesity is a 59.9 per cent and the average risk is a flat 59 per cent. I don't think I am going to be obese any time soon … Carrier status … These are things I can actually print out for my children and be like, don't be an asshole, you might actually have this …

In this edited section of Pandy's autobiological video, she weaves knowledge from the genetic testing into her own story about health and illness. Pandy often interpreted her genetic test findings in light of her own family history: hypertension ran in the family, so she 'sees that one coming'; she was surprised about her decreased risk of diabetes since her maternal grandmother had that; and the decreased risk of melanoma since her father had that. She followed hyperlinks to find out the alleles and markers which made up her results. She wove in and out of describing these findings as susceptibilities and diagnoses, wove between her grandmother's health conditions and her potential future children's traits, between refuting the findings and agreeing with them.

Pandy's narrative style was not unusual in our collection of videos, in the ways she thread in and out of diagnosis/susceptibility, family history and genetic markers. In her video titled 'Exploring the "Me-ome"', Jen McCabe recorded herself looking at her 23andMe results for the first time, two days after receiving notification that they were available. She also oscillated between describing her results as probabilities and certainties, between accepting and refuting the findings. Ataralas (who bought the test because she wanted to see if she 'had the genes for coeliac disease, as well as whatever else I had because, hey, it was on sale and I was curious') thought her 'heart stuff would have been higher', since she had looked up the death certificates of relatives on her mother's side and almost everyone had had heart attacks. In her narrative she also talked about the things she could pass onto her (as yet non-existent) children and the diseases she knew she did and didn't have.

These YouTube narratives correspond to what anthropologist Tim Ingold (2007) refers to as 'wayfaring', the term he uses to describe a line that wanders about. In his book *Lines*, he considers many kinds of lines including the genealogical line, which he theorises quite differently from his anthropological predecessors, as a connection *among and between* generations. Rather than occurring in a sequence, this is a line where ancestors weave and lean over each other, touching at different points. Generations become entangled through a series of interlaced trails, where grandchildren learn stories from and about grandparents that they carry forward in life and so forth, the result being a braid of lines that continually extends as lives proceed. Ingold compares his wayfaring line to the traditional genealogical model adopted in anthropology, whereby attributes such as make-up, character and identity are bestowed via genetic and cultural means, as a form of transmission down which pass, from point to point, person to person, the information for how to live life. This more traditional genealogical line is similar to the linear lines that Kaja Finkler (2005: 1065) discusses in her work on genetics and kin work, for Finkler argues that genetics reinforces the linearity of genealogy and kinship, joining individuals together and disallowing memory lapses and the forgetting of the past.

The YouTube videos on the other hand were filled with lapses and skips, with wayfaring lines of biological inheritance. The YouTubers wove between possible futures, the present and the past, and the results about disease outcomes were read simultaneously as probabilities, certainties, susceptibilities and nothing of much importance. The YouTube narratives reflected, to quote Ingold (2007: 119), the 'narrative interweaving of present and past lives [where] retracing the lines of past lives is the way we proceed along our own'. This was a trans-generational flow in which people and knowledge underwent perpetual formation, made evident in autobiologies through the way in which most people make sense of their world; by telling stories. Autobiologies about DTC genetic testing are, to follow Ingold, a narrative interweaving of past and future states of actual and potential illness, where biologies of the past and imagined future biologies touch, and intermingle with biological practices in the present. Telling such stories involves threading in materials, technologies, information, people and gestures, to name a few.

The cultural geographer Nigel Thrift (2011: 7) argues that the world in which Ingold's wandering wayfaring line exists is being rebuilt out of a field of numbers and calculable coordinates. We also found numbers threaded into the wayfaring line, where biological numbers in the form of genetic markers and alleles (Navon, 2011), as well as comparative percentages and hyperlinks, became part of the autobiology, along with other multifactorial risk factors which are far from genetically deterministic (Hacking, 2006: 91; McGowan *et al.*, 2010: 284). The YouTubers worked both on and off 'script' – their genetic results were created within a 23andMe risk assessment framework (Saukko *et al.*, 2012), yet they contributed their own interpretations following wayfaring lines, accepting and refuting findings according to their own understandings of illness, often using the results to explain what they think they already knew.

These empirical findings resonate with those other anthropological and sociological studies of how individuals knit genetics into their own pre-existing stories of relatedness and perceptions of risk. Anthropologist Margaret Lock and colleagues (2006) have argued that genetic knowledge rarely usurps other forms of understanding, but rather is woven into previously held ideas, discussing notions of blended inheritance, where diseases 'run' in the family. Susan Cox and William McKellin (1999: 628) found that the relevance of genetic risk to individuals is fluid and contingent, with information given higher relevance at certain critical junctures and at other times being much less important. These frameworks of understanding are consistent also with Gubrium and Holstein's (1998) notion of 'biographical work', and how individuals bring medical regimes into their own lives (Felde, 2011). The wayfaring line contributes to this literature by describing how individuals weave intergenerationally, where the threads are braided, allowing room for spaces and other fragments of information to be integrated into one's autobiology and understandings of potential and existing illness, whether these may be genetic markers, percentages, websites or environmental effects.

Stories of playful experimentation and consumption

In the previous sections we documented autobiologies in the form of storytelling about biological practices and narratives which weave biological understandings of illness into family histories and other understandings of disease. As we have stated, these are very different stories from illness narratives. While Lone Frank did have symptoms of and a family history of an illness, depression, her story was not one of the experience of living with a disease but rather a search for her molecular make-up through a series of biological technologies. For the YouTubers, they exhibited a sense of indifference towards the results of their genetic testing, an indifference that was possible because they were not patients. Often in their interpretation of results, they might list the names of diseases, displaying no attachment to them, often not being able to pronounce them or know what they are. The engagements with disease and disease risk seem fleeting and 'playful', the moral responsibility that Arthur Frank (1995: 137) describes in the stories of illness seemingly absent and the kinds of biosocial virtual communities of 'at risk' individuals that Novas and Rose (2000: 508) describe and predict, also missing. The YouTubers were easily distracted, by data visualisations, hyperlinks and the multiple tabs they have open. Lone Frank skipped from one test to another.

These findings fit also with the ways in which users describe themselves in other user studies. For example, in a mixed method study using surveys, interviews and focus groups conducted by anthropologists and other social scientists recruiting through an online genetic testing company, they found in their surveys that users mostly identified as being in good health (Lee *et al.*, 2013). Most participants rated their health as either excellent or very good, indicating that these users did not identify as patients.

In using the word 'playful' to discuss how users engaged with genetic testing services, we draw on the work of Horlick-Jones *et al.* (2007) who describes the playful way in which individuals respond to the interpretive possibilities regarding issues of genetic modification. Horlick-Jones *et al.* (2007: 84–85) incorporate this sense of playfulness, as part of a bricolage of sense-making – a term they take from Irwin (who takes it from Levi-Strauss) – whereby people use, inventively and playfully, whatever comes to hand. This bricolage is evident in a number of ways in the users' stories. In Lone Frank's case, we can see how she tries whatever tests might tell her something about her genetic self, this book following on from a similar accounts of her discovering her 'neuronal self' (2011b). Similarly, the YouTube videos posted about genetic testing were often one or two of many posted by a single individual. The YouTubers video collections may have concerned unboxing other products (a plasma television, a router, a speaker stand), political rallies, music concerts, restaurant reviews or wigs. Self-expression involved not only undergoing genetic testing and consuming/ interpreting/

critiquing/ playing with the results, but also other choices made about the body (hairstyles, tattoos), carefully placed objects in rooms (webcams, posters on bedroom walls) as well as a vast repertoire of other aspects of self-making that defined each YouTuber as both an individual, and as part of a broad set of social groups, telling a story to an 'imagined audience' (Marwick and boyd, 2011a). The stories told by these users could be read as just another online extension of the genetic testing experience, stories to be shared in a participatory environment (John, 2013), and to encourage further participation.

What are the broader conditions of this playful experimentation? The YouTubers were telling stories for themselves and sharing them with their imagined audiences and Lone Frank is doing what journalists do, and telling a good story, involving herself in the science. But both Frank and the YouTubers are also doing work for the company, on a number of levels. First their stories become a form of promotion of the company, a free form of advertising in the same way wearing a branded t-shirt advertises a label. The genetic testers are consumers of a product, their narratives also those of consumption. The YouTuber Zyloga received her spit kit as a 'Materialism Day gift' from her parents, as she says, 'one of the coolest gifts I have ever gotten, way cooler than the bike I was going to ask for instead'. Frank describes 'feeling embarrassed' by her 'passé SNP profile' from deCODEme and wanting to be part of the in-crowd by having the 'latest test'. She writes, 'it almost feels like I'm carrying around a chunky first-generation brick of a Nokia, while everyone else is watching videos on their iPhone 4s' (Frank, 2011a: 138).

Internet platforms such as YouTube has been described as offering a new space for consumers to engage creatively with products and brands and other aspects of consumerism (Pace, 2008: 217). The unboxing videos are most obvious in this aspect, as they document a YouTube practice whereby individuals film themselves opening a box containing a piece of technology, in order to share this experience with others online (Walker, 2009) as well as – semi-didactically – sharing information. The way in which many of the YouTubers discussed product placement of *other* products in their narratives, suggests that they did not consider their videos about 23andMe as explicit advertisements for the company. It would be naïve however, to ignore the consumerist nature of these practices, and the ways in which participatory engagement online, especially concerning genetic testing, is tied into larger economic concerns (see Chapter 4; see also O'Riordan, 2011; Pálsson, 2009).

First, the work of spitting and submitting a saliva sample helps create a valuable database of biological samples for the genetic testing company. Individuals' clinical labour, and the access they give the company to their *in vitro* biology, becomes a biological resource which produces economic value (Mitchell and Waldby, 2010: 339) as we explore further in Chapter 4. There is extensive interplay between genetic testing practices and the production of genomic goods, just as there is interplay between online participation more broadly and the creation of economic value (Goldberg, 2011; O'Riordan, 2010; Proulx *et al.*, 2011). Posting videos online becomes another form of free labour, disguised by altruistic notions such as 'sharing' (John, 2013). Others have also observed and commented on the commodification of illness narratives, including those shared via social media, and the biographical value of these accounts (Mazanderani, Locock and Powell, 2013). The material practices we examine in this paper, documented in the form of autobiology, are thus not only about sense-making and wayfaring, but also about branding and economics.

Potential users and non-users

In addition to examining online material to gain insight into users, we conducted a series of in-depth interviews with people we understood as 'potential users' of DTC genetic tests for psychiatric conditions, that is, people living with a diagnosis or caring for someone living with a diagnosis, in the UK. Interesting to us was that all of these 'potential users' saw themselves as 'potential non-users' with a range of reasons why they would not be interested in purchasing a genetic test for a psychiatric disorder online. We present this material here in order to complement the analysis of online autobiologists, the enthusiastic users of personal genetic testing services, who as we have seen, were far less deterministic in their views of test results than the industry advertising might suggest their users to be. We found in these interviews that, although interested in the potential of genetics particularly with regard to understanding physical illness, there was very little engagement with the idea of genetic testing for understanding themselves. Rather, our respondents were much more interested in finding ways to live best with psychiatric disorders, and were sceptical of commercial interests in testing as well as test efficacy. They expressed more fears about the impacts of genetic testing than excitement or a sense of identity or playfulness.

One area where this was expressed was in predisposition to disease, and what the state of 'patient in waiting' might be like:

> From my point of view I would imagine there is a very long gap between having a predisposition to something and actually having it, and I think it's … having a mental illness anyway I think tends to give people a label and having a label which may be … incorrect isn't probably the right word, but you see what I mean … misapplied, yes, is not going to be helpful.

And from another respondent:

> My fear about people knowing too much is it gives more opportunity for people to come and say 'Oh, you need this, that or the other.' And prescribe treatments ahead of the initial onset of a disorder, which will completely ruin someone's quality of life. Especially in cases where, if you can imagine the future where somebody would have had a perfectly normal life without mental disorder because they had a, say, a 60 per cent chance of developing bipolar, psychotic episode or whatever … they would say, 'Oh, we got to put you on a heavy dose of mood stabilisers to make sure you're safe.'

A number of these respondents were sceptical of what they saw as a lack of transparency with regard to ordering genetic tests from a company over the internet, being involved in a commercial transaction that involved the materiality of their DNA. As one respondent said, 'my DNA in their little jam jar ... Who might own it?'

It was clear from the interviews that there were many reasons why these 'potential users' of DTC genetic tests for psychiatric disorders such as those marketed by several companies were likely to be non-users, and far from sharing the sense of hopefulness and empowerment with which such testing was portrayed, the tests were viewed with fear and distrust.

Conclusion

In this chapter we have discussed a range of different users of genetic testing services, from the users documented in the research of others and the users we studied ourselves, such as the celebrity user and the non-celebrity users posting videos on YouTube, as well as potential users or rather potential non-users. The latter group gave us an interesting perspective on reasons for non-use. The videos and celebrity accounts offered insights into the practices of those engaging in genetic testing, the settings in which this is occurring and the ways in which people are interpreting their results. Among the users we found narratives which we described as autobiologies. Autobiologies differ from illness narratives in that they are not stories about states of sickness and suffering, but are rather narratives of playfulness, possible to those 'in-waiting' who can afford a more casual engagement with the technologies. It may be that the media by which these stories are told, YouTube video for example, invites a more casual performance, an indifference towards illness that may differ from other forms of storytelling, highlighting the importance of context in analysis of these narratives.

We have highlighted the advantage of using the term 'autobiology' to consider these narratives about emerging states of illness ambiguity. Autobiologies draw from and contribute to the world of DTC genetic testing – they become part of the online texts about genetic testing, and the companies themselves are increasingly playing with this format with video competitions and other YouTube related activities, no doubt aware of the conversations their customers are having on this platform. As Ingold (2007: 116) writes, 'making their ways through the tangle of the world, wayfarers grow into its fabric and contribute through their movements to its ever-evolving weave'. The user accounts we studied originate from moments of biological experimentation and consumerism in bedrooms and offices, but as the wayfaring stories which emerge from the interpretation of results show, the stories stretch back into past lives and reach out into imagined biological futures.

Autobiologies are user narratives which form part of a broader shift towards public stories about genetics and other healthcare technologies and experiences, which concern people's exploration and sharing of their own biology (e.g. Abadie, 2010; Duncan, 2009). They are not entirely new ways of telling stories about self, healthcare and technology but they are becoming increasingly ubiquitous. Biological self-testing and monitoring technologies in previous eras also gave rise to narratives that interwove biography with information gained about one's biological being, gleaned from some self-administered technological objects, such as the pregnancy test for example. Autobiologies occur widely across the cultural landscapes of (at least) highly industrialised societies, with an increasing presence of devices allowing us to monitor our biological selves (e.g. blood sugar, heart rate, blood pressure) and to weave these 'data' into our personal narratives. The Quantified Self movement, so named by its guru Gary Wolf in an article in *Wired* magazine (Wolf, 2009), involves the use of self-tracking devices that create data about details such as one's sleep patterns, exercise, food and drink input and output, mood, and an ever-expanding array of data about one's own organism, with the motto 'self-knowledge through numbers' (Wolf, 2009). Self-tracking devices producing personalised data are framed as giving us powerful insight into our true selves, as well as being a means via 'feedback loops' of altering and optimising those selves. It is possible to create and inhabit an ongoing autobiology, narrating every daily ebb and flow, peak and trough, of our biological being. A wearable platform for monitoring physical activity is the Nike+, a shoe cum window into the workings of body and self (see McClusky, 2009).

The possibilities of autobiology continue to expand with the creativity of platform producers. 'Life logging' has become a cultural trope, a form of self-narrative (told not only to selves but to aggregated others, some of whom track with you, compare and respond). According to Lupton:

> As part of these processes, self-trackers interpret 'the numbers' they produce on themselves in certain ways based on how they want the numbers to represent them or underlying assumptions about what they mean. In interpreting their data, self-trackers often negotiate the meanings of what the haptic sensations of their bodies tells them about themselves and what other forms of data reveal. No form of information, whether derived from one's senses or from digital devices, is necessarily taken as authoritative. The skills of interpretation that are part of reflexive self-monitoring are employed in evaluating which data to trust, which to take note of.
>
> (Lupton, forthcoming)

That is, self-tracking data provide the material for interpretation in the storytelling context of one's life.

The possibilities of autobiology expand also with understandings of the human organism associated with changing directions of the life sciences, from neuroscience and its performative imaging, to personal 'microbiome' testing (that is, the para-selves of non-human micro-organisms that inhabit the human body, and tell 'stories' about where and how a particular body, or self, has lived, eaten, drunk, washed, exercised, slept). The company Ubiome, for example, explicitly offers the opportunity to compare oneself with others 'like us' in the sense of having a similar microbiome, via a personal microbiome testing service, not unlike the DTC genetic testing companies, although the biological sampling process is different. The personal bio-sensing device market is growing, we are told, in combination with personal mobile devices and their platforms. Will auto-biologies grow with it?

References

Abadie, R. (2010) *The professional guinea pig: Big pharma and the risky world of human subjects*, Durham, NC: Duke University Press.

Adams, S. (2013) 'Post-panoptic surveillance through healthcare rating sites', *Information, Communication and Society*, vol. 16, no. 2, pp. 215–235.

Akrich, M. (1992) 'The de-scription of technical objects', in W. Bijker and J. Law (eds), *Shaping technology/Building society*, Cambridge, MA: MIT Press, pp. 205–224.

Armstrong, D. (1995) 'The rise of surveillance medicine', *Sociology of Health and Illness*, vol. 17, no. 3, pp. 393–404.

Bennett, J. (2010) *Vibrant matter: A political ecology of things*, Durham, NC: Duke University Press.

boyd, d. (2014) *It's complicated: The social lives of networked teens*, New Haven, CT: Yale University Press.

Chou, W-Y. S., Hunt, Y., Folkers, A. and Augustson, E. (2011) 'Cancer survivorship in the age of YouTube and social media: A narrative analysis', *Journal of Medical Internet Research*, vol. 13, no.1, article e7.

Cox, S. M. and McKellin, W. (1999) '"There's this thing in our family": Predictive testing and the construction of risk for Huntington Disease', *Sociology of Health and Illness*, vol. 21, no. 5, pp. 622–646.

Darnovsky, M. (2008) 'The spitterati and trickle-down genomics', *Mother Jones*, 3 November, available at www.geneticsandsociety.org/article.php?id=4360 (accessed 1 December 2015).

Duncan, D. E. (2009) *Experimental man: What one man's body reveals about his future, your health, and our toxic world*, New York, NY: John Wiley & Sons.

Felde, L. H. (2011) 'Elevated cholesterol as biographical work: Expanding the concept of "biographical disruption"', *Qualitative Sociology Review*, vol. 7, no. 2, pp. 101–120.

Finkler, K. (2005) 'Family, kinship, memory and temporality in the age of the new genetics', *Social Science and Medicine*, vol. 61, pp. 1059–1071.

Frank, A. (1995) *The wounded storyteller: Body, illness, and ethics*, Chicago, IL: University of Chicago Press.

Frank, L. (2011a) *My beautiful genome: Exposing our genetic future, one quirk at a time*, Oxford: Oneworld.

Frank, L. (2011b) *The neurotourist: Postcards from the edge of brain science*, Oxford: Oneworld.

Goldberg, G. (2011) 'Rethinking the public/virtual sphere: the problem with participation', *New Media and Society*, vol. 13, no. 5, pp. 739–754.

Greaves, D. (2000) 'The creation of partial patients', *Cambridge Quarterly of Healthcare Ethics*, vol. 9, no. 1, pp. 23–33.

Gubrium, J. F. and Holstein, J. A. (1998) 'Narrative practice and the coherence of personal stories', *The Sociological Quarterly*, vol. 39, no. 1, pp. 163–187.

Hacking, I. (2006) 'Genetics, biosocial groups and the future of identity', *Daedalus*, Fall, pp. 81–95.

Horlick-Jones, T., Walls, J. and Kitzinger, J. (2007) 'Bricolage in action: Learning about, making sense of, and discussing, issues about genetically modified crops and food', *Health, Risk and Society*, vol. 9, no. 1, pp. 83–103.

Ingold, T. (2007) *Lines: A brief history*, Oxford: Routledge.

John, N. A. (2013) 'Sharing and web 2.0: The emergence of a keyword', *New Media and Society*, vol. 15, no. 2, pp. 167–182.

Kerr, A. (2004) 'Genetics and citizenship', in N. Stehr (ed.), *Biotechnology between commerce and civil society*, New Brunswick, NJ: Transaction Press, pp. 159–174.

Lee, S. S., Vernez, S. L., Ormond, K. E. and Granovetter, M. (2013) 'Attitudes towards social networking and sharing behaviors among consumers of direct-to-consumer personal genomics', *Journal of Personalized Medicine*, vol. 3, no. 4, pp. 275–287.

Lock, M., Freeman, J., Sharples, R. and Lloyd, S. (2006) 'When it runs in the family: Putting susceptibility genes in perspective', *Public Understanding of Science*, vol. 15, no. 3, pp. 277–300.

Lupton, D. (forthcoming) 'You are your data: Self-tracking practices and concepts of data', in S. Selke (ed.), *Lifelogging: Theoretical approaches and case studies about self-tracking*, Sydney: Springer.

McClucsky, M. (2009) 'The Nike experiment: How the shoe giant unleashed the power of personal metrics', *Wired*, 22 June, available at http://archive.wired.com/medtech/health/magazine/17-07/lbnp_nike?currentPage=all (accessed 28 April 2015).

McGowan, M. L., Fishman, J. R. and Lambrix, M. A. (2010) 'Personal genomics and individual identities: Motivations and moral imperatives of early users', *New Genetics and Society*, vol. 29, no. 3, pp. 261–290.

Maher, B. (2011) 'Nature readers flirt with personal genomics: Survey reveals eagerness to use latest DNA technologies', *Nature*, vol. 478, pp. 19–20.

Marwick, A. E. and boyd, d. (2011a) 'I tweet honestly, I tweet passionately: Twitter users, context collapse, and the imagined audience', *New Media and Society*, vol. 13, no.1, pp. 114–133.

Marwick, A. E. and boyd, d. (2011b) 'To see and be seen: Celebrity practice on Twitter', *Convergence: The International Journal of Research into New Media Technologies*, vol. 17, pp. 139–158.

Mazanderani, F., Locock, L. and Powell, J. (2013) 'Biographical value: Towards a conceptualisation of the commodification of illness narratives in contemporary healthcare', *Sociology of Health and Illness*, vol. 35, no. 6, pp. 891–905.

Miller, D. and Sinanan, J. (2013) *Webcam*, Cambridge, UK: Polity Press.

Mitchell, R. and Waldby, C. (2010) 'National biobanks: clinical labor, risk production, and the creation of biovalue', *Science, Technology and Human Values*, vol. 35, no. 3, pp. 330–355.

Navon, D. (2011) 'Genomic designation: how genetics can delineate new, phenotypically diffuse medical categories', *Social Studies of Science*, vol. 41, no. 2, pp. 203–226.

Newman, M. A., Ziebland, S. and Barker, K. (2009) 'Patients' views of a multimedia resource featuring experiences of rheumatoid arthritis: Pilot evaluation of www.healthtalkonline.org', *Health Informatics Journal*, vol. 15, no.2, pp. 147–159.

Nordgren, A. and Juengst, E. T. (2009) 'Can genomics tell me who I am? Essentialistic rhetoric in direct-to-consumer DNA testing', *New Genetics and Society*, vol. 28, no. 2, pp. 157–172.

Novas, C. and Rose, N. (2000) 'Genetic risk and the birth of the somatic individual', *Economy and Society*, vol. 29, no.4, pp. 485–513.

O'Riordan, K. (2010) *Genomes incorporated*, Aldershot: Ashgate.

O'Riordan, K. (2011) 'Writing biodigital life: Personal genomes and digital media', *Biography*, vol. 43, no.1, pp. 119–131.

Oudshoorn, N. and Pinch, T. (2005a) (eds) *How users matter: The co-construction of users and technology*, Cambridge, MA: MIT Press.

Oudshoorn, N. and Pinch, T. (2005b) 'Introduction', in N. Oudshoorn and T. Pinch (eds), *How users matter: The co-construction of users and technology*, Cambridge, MA: MIT Press, pp. 1–25.

Pace, S. (2008) 'YouTube: An opportunity for consumer narrative analysis?', *Qualitative Market Research*, vol. 11, no.2, pp. 213–226.

Pálsson, G. (2009) 'Biosocial relations of production', *Comparative Studies in Society and History*, vol. 51, no.2, pp. 288–313.

Pinker, S. (2009) 'My genome, my self', *The New York Times*, 7 January, available at www.nytimes.com/2009/01/11/magazine/11Genome-t.html?pagewanted=all&_r=0 (accessed 2 September 2015).

Plows, A. and Boddington, P. (2006) 'Troubles with biocitizenship?' *Genomics, Society and Policy*, vol. 2, no.3, pp. 115–135.

Proulx, S., Heaton, L., Choon, M. and Millette, M. (2011) 'Paradoxical empowerment of *produsers* in the context of informational capitalism', *New Review of Hypermedia and Multimedia*, vol. 17, no.1, pp. 9–29.

Rabinow, P. (1996) *Essays on the anthropology of reason*, Princeton, NJ: Princeton University Press.

Raman S. and Tutton, R. (2010) 'Life, science and biopower', *Science, Technology and Human Values*, vol. 35, no.5, pp. 711–734.

Rose, N. (2007) *The politics of life itself: Biomedicine, power, and subjectivity in the twenty-first century*, Princeton, NJ: Princeton University Press.

Rose, N. and Novas, C. (2005) 'Biological citizenship', in A. Ong and S. Collier (eds), *Global assemblages: Technology, politics and ethics as anthropological problems*, Oxford: Blackwell, pp. 439–463.

Rosenberg, C. (2009) 'Managed fear', *The Lancet*, vol. 373, no. 9666, pp. 802–803.

Saukko, P. M., Farrimond, H. R., Evans, P. and Qureshi, N. (2012) 'Beyond beliefs: Risk assessment technologies shaping patients' experiences of heart disease prevention', *Sociology of Health and Illness*, vol. 34, no 4, pp. 560–575.

Shifman, L. (2012) 'An anatomy of a YouTube meme', *New Media and Society*, vol. 14, no. 2, pp. 187–203.

Su, Y., Howard, H. and Borry, P. (2011) 'Users' motivations to purchase direct-to-consumer genome-wide testing: An exploratory study of personal stories', *Journal of Community Genetics*, vol. 2, no. 3, pp. 135–146.

Syed-Abdul, S., Fernandez-Luque, L., Jian, W. S., Li, Y. C., Crain, S., Hsu, M. H., Wang, Y. C., Khandregzen, D., Chuluunbaatar, E., Nguyen, P. A. and Liou, D. M (2013) 'Misleading health-related information promoted through video-based social media: Anorexia on YouTube', *Journal of Medical Internet Research*, vol. 15, no. 2, article e30.

Thrift, N. (2011) 'Lifeworld Inc: And what to do about it', *Environment and Planning D: Society and Space*, vol. 29, pp. 5–26.

Tian, Y. (2010) 'Organ donation on web 2.0: Content and audience analysis of organ donation videos on YouTube', *Health Communication*, vol. 25, no. 3, pp. 238–246.

Timmermans, S. and Buchbinder, M. (2010) 'Patients-in-waiting', *Journal of Health and Social Behavior*, vol. 51, no. 4, pp. 408–423.

Walker, T. (2009) 'Unboxing: The new geek porn', *The Independent*, 14 January, available at www.independent.co.uk/life-style/gadgets-and-tech/features/unboxing-the-new-geek-porn-1333955.html (accessed 1 December 2015).

Wohlsen, M. (2011) *Biopunk: DIY scientists hack the software of life*, New York: Current.

Wolf, G. (2009) 'Know thyself: Tracking every facet of life, from sleep to mood to pain', *Wired*, 22 June, available at http://archive.wired.com/medtech/health/magazine/17-07/lbnp_knowthyself (accessed 25 April 2015).

Wyatt, S. (2005) 'Non-users also matter: the construction of users and non-users of the Internet', in N. Oudshoorn and T. Pinch (eds), *How users matter: The co-construction of users and technology*, Cambridge, MA: MIT Press, pp.67–79.

Yoo, J. H. and Kim, J. (2011) 'Obesity in the new media: A content analysis of obesity videos on YouTube', *Health Communication*, vol. 27, no.1, pp. 86–97.

3   Professionals

In this chapter we examine some implications of DTC genetic testing for a set of key actors, healthcare professionals. We focus on the case of genetic counselling for several reasons. First, the DTC genetic testing industry largely operates out of the US, where genetic counselling is well established as a healthcare profession. Second, a key element of consumers receiving genetic test results outside of the clinic was the lack of direct involvement of 'gatekeeper' healthcare professionals, not only physicians but also genetic counsellors. Third, we were fascinated by the response of the DTC genetic testing industry to critiques that healthcare professionals were not involved, and how genetic counselling was involved in the response of a number of companies. We are interested in this reflexivity, as well as in the profession itself.

Early critiques of the DTC genetic testing industry focused on the reconfiguration of 'traditional' relations among actors entailed in the ordering and receipt of genetic tests, by offering personal genetic information directly to consumers over the internet rather than that information being accessed by consumers/patients via a healthcare professional. (In Chapter 2 we discuss users, and that users are co-constructors of technologies. We identify healthcare professionals as users, as discussed below, and in this chapter examine aspects of that co-construction.) That is, while direct access to one's 'personal' genetic information has been a key marketing point of consumer genetics products often described as an empowering 'right', a common point of concern has been how individuals may (mis)understand, (mis)interpret and potentially be harmed by the genetic information that they are provided from genetic tests if these are not ordered through a healthcare professional (American Congress of Obstetricians and Gynecologists, 2008; Couzin, 2008; Hudson et al., 2007; NSGC, 2010a). Specifically, DTC genetic testing companies have been criticised for providing genetic information outside of the more traditional clinical context in which such information is usually conveyed, which includes the presumed safeguards afforded by genetic counselling (Hennen, Sauter and Van Den Cruyce, 2010; Nuffield Council on Bioethics, 2010; Udesky, 2010; Wade and Wilfond, 2006: 285).

More broadly, some scholars have observed that genetic information and genome sequencing technologies are transforming and reconfiguring the boundaries between patients and consumers, between research and clinical practice, and between public and private domains (and raising new ethical questions; see for example Kaye *et al.*, 2010). It is less frequently observed that these roles are themselves being reframed, given new meaning, not by 'new' technologies but by their users, including DTC genetic testing companies, healthcare professionals, patients and consumers. In this chapter, we argue that it is as important to attend to the different ways in which these actors are being framed and positioned (or are framing and positioning themselves), as it is to attend to shifting boundaries between them. This framing and positioning may, as we find in the case of genetic counsellors, involve shifts in core tenets of the profession beyond technical expertise, such as engagement with a family over time, rather than a one-time interaction with an individual regarding interpretation of their test results.

We are arguing for attention to the co-production of users and technologies not only in the DTC genetic testing industry, but also in other areas where information and genome sequencing technologies are viewed as transformational. We suggest that such co-production may involve how actors are positioned with regard to one another, and the nature of relationships involved. For example, both healthcare professionals and patients are framed as consumers, in various ways and by at least some DTC genetic testing companies, the notion of consumers being associated with a specific set of assumptions regarding motivation and relationships with others. Being so framed, however, healthcare professionals and patients have ambiguous relationships to clinical spaces in which healthcare professional/patient relationships are traditionally located (see for example McGowan *et al.*, 2014). As we have noted elsewhere (Wyatt *et al.*, 2013), this shifting configuration relies on and has implications for trust – trust in healthcare professions, trust in the internet, trust in science, and trust in institutions – as well as the distribution of expertise within medical systems.

In this chapter, we address questions about shifting roles and boundaries among variously positioned actors by focusing on healthcare professionals, a type of actor frequently perceived to be disrupted, displaced or reconfigured by the selling of personal genomic information directly to consumers via the internet. That is, we focus on the co-production of healthcare professionals and the DTC genetic testing industry. 'Healthcare professional' is a heterogeneous category, comprising general practitioners, specialists, genetic counsellors, nurses, 'in house' as well as 'external' providers; here we examine genetic counselling. We focus attention on healthcare professionals in co-producing possibilities of social relations opened by genetics going online, asking, as did Diana Forsythe (1996) years ago, whether this is 'new bottles, old wine'?

Much of the research examining the DTC genetic testing industry assumes a shared understanding of DTC genetic testing as the selling of genetic tests to the public unmediated by a physician (e.g. Hennen, Sauter and Van Den Cruyce, 2010; Hock *et al.*, 2011; McGowan *et al.*, 2010; Richards, 2010). In this analysis, we define DTC genetic testing as the offer (advertising or selling) of genetic testing services to consumers, whom we define as the general public, patients *and* physicians. We include physicians in our definition of consumers as many of the genetic testing products are marketed either directly to doctors, or to doctors and the public/patients simultaneously (it is important to note that physicians and scientists are also involved in this arena by working directly for the industry; raising another set of issues about the stretching of clinical relations and of trust). The involvement of doctors as consumers of DTC genetic testing is also heterogeneous, and includes those who directly order the test, those who sign forms supplied by their patients, and those with relationships with companies who may mediate between test providers and patients. Others have recognised the trend towards advertisement of DTC genetic testing to doctors, and have noted that this, as well as the involvement of in-house physicians within these companies, is an ethically problematic development in this industry (McGowan *et al.*, 2014; Howard and Borry, 2012). Michelle McGowan and colleagues (2014) specifically have questioned whether physicians ordering tests on behalf of consumers are providing a professional 'gatekeeping' service or actually offering independent advice and interpretation of genetic results. We also are interested in how these actor positions play out, and are related to each other as well as to 'traditional' professional and clinical relationships.

This broader definition of consumer is important in considering the evolving role of healthcare professionals in the DTC genetic testing arena, and we discuss this issue further in relation to physicians' engagement with genetic counsellors employed within the industry. It is worth reiterating that our definition of DTC genetic testing encompasses a wide variety of commercial enterprises, including well-established genetic testing services that specialise in monogenetic and rare genetic diseases and newer companies offering susceptibility testing for a large number of common complex health conditions alongside traits and other non-health related information.

This chapter illustrates these concerns with empirical insights from our examination of genetic counselling in the context of DTC genetic testing. Specifically, we conducted discourse analysis of ways in which the healthcare profession of genetic counselling has been represented on DTC genetic testing websites, blogs and other online material, and ways in which members of the genetic counselling profession have responded in these fora (see Appendix A for more details). Genetic counselling is a healthcare profession that has developed specifically to inform and counsel patients about genetic testing, test results, and the meaning of those results for patients and their relatives. The provision of genetic counselling with online genetic testing can be seen to challenge some of the traditional roles of counsellors, and to provide opportunities for new roles. Offering genetic testing (itself a heterogeneous category) without the requirement of meeting with a genetic counsellor or other healthcare professional means that consumers do not have the opportunity to engage this way of increasing their knowledge and understanding of the test results, including possible consequences of the tests for themselves, their relatives, and their health (Howard and Borry, 2008). We contextualise the discussion by considering the complexity of genetic information provided by DTC genetic testing, the mediating role of the internet in counselling, and potential conflicts of interest of genetic counsellors enrolled by companies (see for example, American Congress of Obstetricians and Gynecologists, 2008;

European Society of Human Genetics, 2010; Genetics and Public Policy Center, 2006). The chapter closes with reflections about issues raised by internet technologies being used in telegenetic and other clinical settings, and the broader question of what these developments might mean for healthcare professionals.

Genetic counselling online: co-production of users and technologies

Critiques of genetic testing products being advertised and sold on the internet have been accompanied by calls for the provision of pre- and post-test counselling within the industry (American College of Medical Genetics Board of Directors, 2004; American Congress of Obstetricians and Gynecologists, 2008; Jordens, Kerridge and Samuel, 2009). Here we examine how the industry and other actors have responded to these concerns, and with what implications for consumers, the product, and healthcare professionals. The involvement of healthcare professionals including genetic counsellors was a response to criticisms of how the DTC industry initially configured its genetic testing product as 'personal', for individuals to access and act upon on their own, outside of clinical contexts (McGowan *et al.*, 2014).

Accompanying calls for genetic counselling to be provided with DTC genetic tests, concerns have been raised about how and with what implications such counselling would be provided. For example, will consumers be influenced in their beliefs about genetic testing by advertisements, and by the arguably exaggerated (Hock *et al.*, 2011) claims found on DTC genetic testing websites (Wade and Wilfond, 2006)?

Concerns have also been raised about genetic counsellors taking on the role of making preventative health-related recommendations, such as behaviour or lifestyle changes, based on DTC genetic testing results. This concern is related to the fact that DTC genetic testing results are often based on, or reference, genome-wide association study (GWAS) data for common conditions, which provide relatively small contributions to predictions of disease risk (O'Daniel, 2010), and are often not well replicated. Some tests are based on genome-wide single nucleotide polymorphism (SNP) panels. Health behaviour recommendations from these predictions are often similar to those for healthy living in general (Leighton *et al.*, 2012), but other recommendations could include those with significant impact, such as reproductive decisions.

It has also been suggested that preventative health advice in this context sits problematically with non-directive genetic counselling (Rees *et al.*, 2006), a practice that is being reframed in the context of health-promoting medical settings (Koch and Nordahl Svendsen, 2005). There is a general concern about limited family history taking. The question has also been raised whether DTC genetic testing falls within genetic counsellors' scope of practice, particularly where it is concerned with common complex diseases rather than single gene, Mendelian inheritance conditions, new or otherwise (Clarke and Thirlaway, 2011; Hock *et al.*, 2011). Whereas genetic counsellors traditionally assist clients to evaluate personal and familial consequences of particular decisions based on genetic risk information, the broader activity of health risk assessment potentially associated with DTC genetic testing tests may re-focus counsellors' attention and activities more toward promoting or achieving behavioural changes. However, some have argued that the genetic counselling profession needs to embrace developments occurring in DTC genetic testing, recommending that counsellors use their expertise in genetics productively in order to provide services to DTC genetic testing customers and their healthcare providers (O'Daniel, 2010; Weaver and Pollin, 2012). In either scenario, the profession is seen to be responding to how they are positioned relative to other actors and to technologies in the arena, both by the companies and by critics.

The provision of genetic counselling within the DTC genetic testing industry has thus been a controversial issue, one that may be challenging many of the traditional roles of counsellors. Following the National Society of Genetic Counselors (NSGC) and the American Board of Genetic Counseling (ABGC), we define genetic counselling as providing information and support to individuals and families at risk of genetic disease (NSGC, 2011; ABGC, 2009). We use the definition provided by these American organisations considering that most websites we analysed were registered in the US. According to the NSGC and ABGC, counselling includes interpretation of family, medical and psychosocial histories in order to assess genetic risk, as well as the provision of modified information, in response to verbal and nonverbal cues, in a 'culturally responsive' and 'non-coercive' manner (ABGC, 2009: 2) that promotes decision making and guides prevention and disease management.

Although we recognise that the distinction between 'traditional' and 'non-traditional' genetic counselling is now blurred (Finucane, 2012: 3), central tenets of genetic counselling are missing from the DTC genetic testing context, particularly the use of strong interpersonal skills and emotional intelligence through face-to-face counselling (Finucane, 2012), with time provided to explore patient values and life experiences, where knowledge about the individual and family is brought into conjunction with pedigrees and other shards of information collected through the counselling encounter (Featherstone *et al.*, 2006). However, in the study by McGowan and colleagues (2014) previously cited, some *physicians* ordering tests on behalf of patients claimed to have developed strong relationships with company-based counsellors upon whom they relied for information.

Professional roles and boundaries may be disrupted by technological change, as Petrakaki *et al.* (2011) highlight in their study of how communication technology is shaping the profession of community pharmacists in England. Although most genetic counsellors work in clinical or hospital settings (NSGC, 2011), genetic counsellors have also been working in the commercial context for some time, such as in pharmaceutical, insurance and biotech companies (the NSGC Professional Status Survey reported that 9 per cent of genetic counsellors worked in commercial laboratories and 20 per cent worked in other non-clinical settings, including commercial industry) (NSGC, 2010b). DTC genetic testing presents a new context for genetic counselling however, and the diversity of opinions mentioned above reflects the importance of this industry in potentially shifting roles within the profession. Perhaps the most important point, looking back to the time of our analysis, is not where members of the profession work, but ways in which some of the normative aspects of the professional role have shifted, with a re-positioning of relationships within the healthcare arena.

Not that genetic counselling has not undergone shifts in the past. The history of genetic counselling has been continually shaped by responses to technological advances (Kenen, 1997; Pagon, 2002), as well as broader shifts in understandings of obligations and expectations pertaining to lay/professional relations. The profession has undergone previous shifts in terms of roles and boundaries (Novas and Rose, 2000). In the 1950s, the profession started to move from a strategy of public education towards an emphasis on non-directive counselling, with an emphasis on the client's autonomy in decision making, in order to distance counselling from prior eugenic practices. In the 1970s, genetic counselling became more focused on the communication of genetic risk, with another more recent shift taking place due to the pre-symptomatic testing of the self-directed, self-responsible client (Novas and Rose, 2000). This shift points to a wider re-positioning of relationships, and expectations regarding the nature of relationships, within the healthcare arena, of which genetic counselling is a part. Kenen (1997) documents shifts that occurred in the American genetic counselling profession in the 1990s, in part as a result of healthcare restructuring according to principles of managed care. It has been suggested that the increasing emphasis in clinical settings on genetic predisposition to common complex diseases is instituting another professional shift (Pagon, 2002). We situate DTC genetic testing within this historical context, with responses to technology and positioning of the profession by a range of actors, engendering another shift in the continually evolving genetic counselling profession, prompting reflection upon what it means to be a genetic counsellor in this 'genomic era' (Guttmacher and Collins, 2003).

Considering the emphasis of many European and North American medical organisations on the need for genetic counselling in DTC genetic testing, there has been surprisingly little empirical investigation of the representations of genetic counselling in the DTC genetic testing industry. Hennen, Sauter and Van Den Cruyce (2010), and authors of a recent publication from the Genetics and Public Policy Center (2011) document the presence of genetic counselling provided by DTC genetic testing companies, but provide little analysis. In the small amount of genetic counselling literature concerning DTC genetic testing at the time of our analysis (e.g. O'Daniel, 2010), there has been little acknowledgement of genetic counsellors' employment by DTC genetic testing companies, a silence which we may read as 'boundary work' or demarcation (Nancarrow and Borthwick, 2005). This is surprising given the concerns that many medical organisations have expressed about potential conflicts that may arise when genetic counsellors are employed by the genetic testing industry (American Congress of Obstetricians and Gynecologists, 2008; European Society of Human Genetics, 2010; Genetics and Public Policy Center, 2006).

In this analysis, we are interested in how genetic counselling is *represented* by the DTC genetic testing websites, examining the types of genetic testing products with which counselling is offered, the forms of counselling offered and the roles attributed to counsellors. We recognise that these relationships and representations are likely continually shifting, and provide an analysis of what we found during our study. We do not profess to make any claims about how genetic counselling *sessions* are conducted in the DTC genetic testing setting, but rather examine the *representation* of genetic counselling online, which is important when considering how this market is taking shape and the potential implications for professional boundaries and roles. We analyse how the critiques of the lack of involvement of genetic counsellors in DTC genetic testing are being played out online.

More specifically, we critically explore how genetic counselling expertise is represented on these websites, as well as in other online material such as blogs (the methods through which we conducted this study, our sample and procedures, and our analytic approaches are detailed in Appendix A). We argue that, at the time of the analysis, there seemed to be shifts underway in how genetic counsellors' professional roles were being represented. We consider how these emerging roles sit with more traditional aspects of genetic counselling. We also argue that genetic counsellors have an important part to play in how the DTC genetic testing market is taking shape (that is, in co-production), particularly in terms of the mediation of testing, counsellors' engagement with physicians, and the entrepreneurial activities of some genetic counsellors, as many of these practices are moving DTC genetic testing more firmly toward medical products and information (with implications for how regulators have perceived the industry's activities, among other implications). We end by broadening out our discussion to healthcare professions more broadly.

Representations of genetic counselling by direct-to-consumer genetic testing companies

Our analysis found that representations of genetic counselling in the DTC genetic testing industry were shifting from some of the traditional roles and tenets as described above. Of the 20 companies we identified, 14 did not provide genetic counselling (although several, such as EasyDNA, suggested that customers pursue genetic counselling), five did provide counselling (DeCODEme, GeneDx, Lineagen, Navigenics and Pathway Genomics) and one company offered what we have referred to below as 'independent' counselling (23andMe). Several of these companies claimed to be the only genetic testing company to offer genetic counselling as part of the testing service, perhaps representing the state of flux of the industry at the time of our analysis, and the relationships configured around it. Nonetheless, our analysis found that two of these companies had been providing counselling services for over ten years, whereas two companies started offering counselling in 2008, shortly after the launch of the best known companies and the initiation of critiques of the industry. The websites varied in how they presented their genetic counselling services, with some listing the service in 'FAQs', and others promoting counselling prominently under 'what we offer' or 'about us'.

All counsellors represented on these websites were women, except for two men employed at GeneDx. Genetic counselling was available by phone, Skype or email – what some researchers refer to as 'telegenetics' (O'Daniel, 2010). Three companies offered counselling pre- and post-test, and three offered counselling post-test only. Of the companies offering genetic counselling, all websites were registered in the US, except for DeCODEme.

Some of the companies we studied did not consider themselves to be 'direct-to-consumer' because a physician was required to order the test. We have included these companies in our group nonetheless, because as discussed earlier, we include physicians in our definition of consumers of DTC genetic testing. Three of the DTC genetic testing companies administered blogs which we also analysed wherever they discussed genetic counselling: these were the Navigenics Blog, The Spittoon (23andMe) and the Pathway Genomics blog. We also analysed four blogs which were not administered by DTC genetic testing companies: DNA Exchange, Wellsphere, PsychCentral and the Western States Genetics blog.

Models of genetic counselling provision

From our analysis of this online material we identified four representations of genetic counselling provision in the market: the integrated counselling product, discretionary counselling, independent counselling, and product advice. Each of these is described below. (In this section, all quotations are from analysed web material.)

- *Integrated counselling*: the genetic counselling service was marketed as an integral part of the genetic testing product, as in the case of GeneDx. GeneDx had been providing genetic counselling for over 10 years, as part of their genetic testing service specialising in rare hereditary disorders. This model of genetic counselling provision closely resembles the more 'traditional' role of genetic counselling. By being integral to the testing product, genetic counselling is not provided at the discretion of the consumer. Rather, determination of test appropriateness, and personal interpretation, are represented as part of the testing process, following a clinical services model. That is, the activities take place outside traditional clinical spaces, but the activities themselves are represented as similar.
- *Discretionary counselling*: the consumer chooses whether or not to contact the DTC genetic testing company's genetic counsellor, for counselling about their own or their patient's test results. Companies varied in how prominently they advertised this service: Navigenics claimed that 'genetic counselling from a qualified professional is a critical part of the genetic testing experience', and Pathway Genomics advertises counsellors in their panel of 'our experts', while DeCODEme mentions genetic counselling only briefly in their FAQ section and in sample reports.
- *Independent counselling*: a service that is offered by an external company. In our group of sites, two companies – 23andMe and DeCODEme – offered

genetic counselling in this way, both through InformedDNA. Independent counselling is a sub-type of discretionary counselling, where the consumer chooses to access the service. Independent counselling is consonant with 23andMe and DeCODEme's empowerment framework that emphasises individual genetic information as a right and consumer choice. 23andMe stated that they deliberately 'engaged' InformedDNA genetic counsellors who are 'trained in 23andMe's unique reports and processes', in order to 'ensure that the information our customers receive is completely objective'. In their blog, Spittoon, a post declared that by doing this the company is adhering to European Society of Human Genetics recommendations that counselling is provided independently of the company.

- *Product advice*: a form of genetic counselling that concerns information provision about the test for sale, which in some circumstances can be seen to be very similar to traditional pre-test counselling. For example, on the Navigenics blog, genetic counsellors are described as helping in the decision about whether testing is appropriate. Product advice may also be given to physicians. One GeneDx genetic counsellor saw herself as playing a vital role in keeping clinics up to date on test offerings.

Genetic counselling roles

Interrelated with various models of genetic counselling provision by the DTC genetic testing companies was the representation of the roles of genetic counsellors. In general, genetic counsellors were represented on the DTC genetic testing websites as personal genetics experts. They were represented as being constantly 'on-call', with websites advertising 'unlimited access', counsellors' availability 'seven days a week', where they were ready 'to help you at any time'. The counsellors' professional knowledge was emphasised through markers such as board certification, ethical guidelines, hyperlinks to well-respected websites such as the National Society of Genetic Counsellors and scientific research. The genetic counsellors' expertise was evident in various, overlapping roles as genetics educator, mediator, lifestyle/health adviser, risk interpreter and entrepreneur:

- *The genetics educator*: the genetic counsellor was represented on a number of sites as having a role in the education of the general (pre-symptomatic, genetically curious) consumer about genetics and the genetic testing product, through the provision of web-based information or pre-test counselling. Genetic counsellors were also represented as having an important role in the education of healthcare providers about genetic testing, positioning other healthcare providers as a specific type of user. For example, Lineagen offered genetic counselling services primarily as an informational service for physicians. Navigenics genetic counsellors were defined as 'trained healthcare professionals that specialize in personal genomics ... dedicated to providing you with the most accurate information to help you, your family, and even your doctor'. Pathway Genomics genetic counsellors were represented as there for when 'a physician or staff member is in need of assistance with clinical information, report interpretation or general customer service'. One genetic counsellor regards this as a shift into physician education, asking on the DNA Exchange blog, 'will we move from being educators of patients to being educators of health professionals?'

- *The mediator*: in many ways part of their educational role, the genetic counsellor on some of the analysed sites was also represented as a mediator between the customer and the physician. A good example was found in the genetic counselling service offered by Navigenics, where their counsellors could help the customer 'determine what to focus on with your doctor – or even speak to your doctor directly if he or she has questions'. The genetic counsellor can also be viewed as a mediator between the customer and the DTC genetic testing company, through their online or phone interactions.

- *The lifestyle/health adviser*: the genetic counsellor was represented as offering advice about lifestyle and health behaviour change concerning a range of complex and rare illnesses as a result of the DTC genetic testing results. Lineagen claimed to offer 'counseling to promote informed choices and adaptation to the risk or condition', and that their counsellors helped families to understand 'what may happen in the future and what treatment or management options are available … [and make] adjustments to the condition and choose courses of action that are best for the children and their families'. (Lineagen has since replaced genetic counselling with a flow diagram and other tools to guide parents and physicians through diagnosis, one step of which includes genetic testing – leading to an assessment of whether a concern should trigger a chain of diagnosis leading events. Their First Step genetic test is described as integrated with genetic testing and counselling.) Navigenics offered to help consumers to integrate information from their test results into their lives, and DeCODEme offered 'counseling to help patients understand what their test results mean for their future health'.

- *The risk interpreter*: the genetic counsellor was represented on websites as a specialist, an expert in risk interpretation. In general, risk interpretation is based principally on the consumers' genomic information obtained from the genetic test. There was no mention of the potentially unspecific or uncertain nature of information provided by DTC genetic testing on the websites we analysed or of the difficulties interpreting genetic information without the context of a detailed family history.

- *The entrepreneur*: a number of genetic counsellors have founded websites which provide telegenetics services, and have been advocates for the important role of genetic counselling in DTC genetic testing. For example, US-based Jordanna Joaquina is a genetic counsellor who founded AccessDNA (renamed Inherited Health, which was subsequently bought by InformedDNA). AccessDNA was represented as 'a leading online consumer resource for genetics', which educated and directed people towards testing services and counselling services. In a guest post for the DNA Exchange blog, Joaquina stated that 'in this brave new world of personalized medicine, I imagine that every person will have their own personal genetic counsellor'.

Genetic counsellors were represented on the websites and blogs we analysed as performing in some or a combination of these roles. The kinds of roles for genetic counsellors on each website generally aligned with the company's targeted consumer, whether this was a proactive customer, patient, carrier or healthcare provider. (In a 'traditional' genetic counselling session a carrier may be considered a patient, but this is not necessarily the case in DTC genetic testing.)

Concerns expressed by interview respondents

We were interested to find that the traditional role of healthcare providers as mediators of genetic information was expected by many of our interview respondents, who assumed this would be necessary, as the information could be 'dangerous' as well as difficult to understand. That is, healthcare providers were seen as both interpreters of the science and as providing psychosocial support. For example, one respondent focused on the different nature of the relationship between a patient and healthcare provider, and that of a customer and a company providing a service, noting the different interests and expectations involved in the different kinds of relationships. It is these kinds of boundary shifts to which we wish to call attention in this analysis, rather than the specific issue of whether complex information is adequately understood. The expectation below concerns the need for support:

> Well, I think there is something to be said for the argument ... in relation to empowerment. Yes, I do think that people are made stronger by information, but I think that that information needs to be contextualised and they need to be supported around the choices that result from it, because it is rarely going to come to them in a way that makes actions completely clear ... So, I think it ... has virtues, but I'm more worried about the direct-to-consumer testing in a vacuum however valiant the endeavours the companies make to try to support people. The commercial realities are that they will have to serve quite a lot of customers to be able to make money and making money is their main objective, rather than supporting people in distress.

New roles for genetic counsellors

In the analysis presented here, we have identified various ways in which the healthcare role of genetic counselling has been represented on the websites of companies offering genetic testing directly to consumers. Many of these roles are emerging as a result of genetic counsellors' involvement in the direct-to-consumer genetic testing industry. Changes in professional roles are taking place within a broader context of ongoing changes in genetic testing processes, biomedical research, genetic result interpretation, and structuring and uses of the internet.

The commercialisation of counselling on the internet, the increasing complexity of the genetic information these internet counsellors are dealing with, and the opening of spaces allowing emerging relations among actors, are contributing to shifts in the profession itself.

While the DTC genetic testing industry is heterogeneous, we can nonetheless make some general claims about how genetic counselling has been represented in the direct-to-consumer genetic testing field. First, the internet as a platform for representation and communication allows the possibility of ambiguity and play with traditional roles, and shifting boundaries of the profession, its practice and expertise. We would want to emphasise however, that the shifts we identify should be understood in terms of agency and temporality, and not as determined by the technology of the internet. Second, shifts in roles assumed by various actors – users, producers, mediators, otherwise – are only partly visible through the ways they are represented by companies. Third, one aspect of the practice of genetic counsellors working in the context of direct to consumer genetic testing that does appear to have shifted quite visibly is the way in which they communicate with clients (consumers, patients, other healthcare professionals). The genetic counsellors on the sites we analysed were in communication with individual consumers either through email or by telephone, rather than face-to-face. Unlike the use of the telephone and internet to reach remote or hard to reach patients – how telegenetics is most commonly used (Abrams and Geier, 2006; Stalker *et al.*, 2006; Zilliacus *et al.*, 2010) – the service is potentially available for all DTC genetic testing consumers, regardless of their geographic location or ability to attend face-to-face sessions. Mediation of the counselling session through telephone and email also challenges genetic counsellors' abilities to read non-verbal cues, and to engage in emotive, embodied interaction (Arribas-Ayllon, Sarangi and Clarke, 2012), traditionally often in a relational context with other family members (Hawkins and Ho, 2012). Various internet platforms also meant that genetic counselling provision and expertise sat alongside other forms of genetic interpretation such as information sheets and online forums available to consumers. These alternative forms of interpretation could be used by consumers to find out risk information, to discuss the implications of their results and to locate further resources. Most importantly for this analysis, genetic counsellors' roles were represented as changing shape, with shifting relationships to other actors promoted on the DTC genetic testing websites. These roles included ways in which counsellors educate physicians and provide product and lifestyle advice, both of which we explore in more detail below.

Physician education

While genetic counsellors have traditionally educated patients and families about genetics, the representation of genetic counsellors employed by the DTC genetic testing industry as genetic educators for physicians appears to be changing as a result of its relationship to the DTC genetic testing product. A precursor to this may be the emphasis that earlier genetic testing companies, such as Myriad, placed on physician education. Myriad Genetics has been offering a commercial BRACAnalysis genetic susceptibility test for hereditary breast cancer since 1996 and is often seen as a forerunner to the large number of DTC genetic testing companies now in operation (Matloff and Caplan, 2008). Myriad invested heavily in patient and physician education, providing extensive online resources and supporting Continuing Medical Education programs for physicians (Williams-Jones and Graham, 2003). The training of doctors in genetics and genetic testing is a delicate issue for genetic counsellors, considering their maintenance of professional identity and boundaries (Kenen, 1997; Skirton *et al.*, 2010).

Product advice

Closely related to their role in physician education is the genetic counsellor's role in providing product advice to healthcare providers and other consumers. The limited training that doctors receive in genetics (Powell *et al.*, 2012) and the requirement for physicians to order the tests in some circumstances at least partly explains why genetic counsellors are represented as becoming involved in providing product advice to consumers. While 47 per cent of hypothetical users of DTC genetic testing in an early study were confident that physicians have enough knowledge to interpret the test (McGuire *et al.*, 2009), research has shown that doctors in fact have very little knowledge of genetics, which leads some to claim that doctors are likely to 'mishandle, misinterpret, and misadvise these patients on what is one of the most important pieces of medical information they will ever receive' (Matloff and Caplan, 2008: 7). For a variety of reasons, some companies are moving or have moved towards a model whereby physicians must order the test (Howard and Borry, 2012). The DTC genetic testing industry could thus be seen as being reliant upon doctors being knowledgeable of genetics and the genetic tests. However, the most striking finding from McGowan and colleagues' 2014 study of clinicians involved in a direct to provider mode with genetic testing companies was that they largely relied on the companies themselves for expertise in interpreting genetic information to their patients in ways that were meaningful for health. As explained in their paper:

> Virtually all of the information study participants used to explain genetic risk susceptibilities to patients came directly from partnering commercial laboratories–through training programs to familiarize clinicians with commercial products and services, pre-test advice on the appropriateness of testing, and/or *ad hoc* counseling by staff genetic counselors to help clinicians interpret test results.
>
> (McGowan *et al.*, 2014: 4)

Just as pharmaceutical representatives have an important role to play in educating physicians about new products (Martin, 2006; Prosser and Walley, 2006) – what Oldani (2004: 334) referred to as 'the art of selling without selling' – genetic counsellors working in the DTC genetic testing industry may have a role in

educating these potential consumers about genetic testing products. This raises a number of questions regarding how relationships among various players in the arena are being configured (actively), and how visible they are (and to whom).

Lifestyle/health behaviour advice

The type of genetic information that is provided by DTC genetic testing differs from the monogenetic information for which genetic counsellors have traditionally been trained. This means that more traditional roles for genetic counsellors, such as risk interpretation and prevention strategies, are, we argue, taking on new forms, as genetic counsellors may be called upon to interpret an ambiguous product that provides information about a large number of genetic associations for complex diseases, based on controversial studies of specific populations, which provide probabilities that are very similar to population risk. One result of this shift, as we observed on the websites, and as O'Daniel (2010) has also noted, is that in dealing with DTC genetic testing results, genetic counsellors are represented as moving towards the provision of preventive health and lifestyle advice about complex disorders, based on small differences in risk.

Some genetic counsellors, writing in blogs, have recognised that these activities are 'non-traditional', with a GeneDx counsellor commenting that 'having genetic counsellors work outside their traditional roles, ensures we will have well informed professionals in these new areas of growth, that benefits not only doctors and counsellors, but also patients and families' (Waltho, 2011). Another counsellor asks, in the same blog, 'in a world ... described as "woefully unprepared" for the era of genomic medicine now approaching with all the subtlety and control of a locomotive off the tracks, the question lingers: where will we find ourselves, in this new landscape?' (Hercher, 2009). Some of the roles that we have identified here have also been recognised by other researchers, and could be considered activities that many genetic counsellors engage in, in some form. For example, Wade and Wilfond (2006: 291) have gestured towards genetic counsellors' roles in educating physicians, nurses and health educators, while Zilliacus *et al.* (2010) point out that genetic counsellors also facilitate communication between patients and clinicians. Hennen, Sauter and Van Den Cruyce (2010) have wondered whether genetic counsellors working in the DTC genetic testing industry are merely facilitating sales transactions. More generally, the 'non-traditional' role of genetic counsellors working in the private sector and concerning communication technologies was also identified by Kenen (1997) in the late 1990s. While the roles we identified in our analysis may not be completely new roles for genetic counsellors, we argue that they are shifting roles within the context of DTC genetic testing, where actors are actively responding to the novelty of the spaces for social relations opened in the DTC genetic testing arena.

The emerging roles (or nuanced shifts) for genetic counsellors represented on the websites are implicitly aligned with and referenced to representations of 'traditional' forms of genetic counselling on the websites. This occurs predominantly through the use of images that show face-to-face counselling sessions, with many counsellors emphasising their clinical experience in their online personal profiles. We argue that this representation is a crucial aspect of the genetic counselling product provided by DTC genetic testing companies, as these 'traditional' images reinforce the genetic test as having clinical significance, thus potentially strengthening consumer trust in the product. We recognise that these representations are temporally located, but the ways in which the healthcare profession of genetic counselling has shifted, if in nuanced ways, while retaining elements of trust from more traditional incarnations suggests areas for further research with other healthcare professionals and the social relations made visible (or not) in the personal genomics arena. This is particularly important where activities become blurred (as in blurring of the activities, and roles, of consumption and research). We are not the first to notice that DTC genetic testing includes ambiguous products situated in a grey area between recreation or entertainment, and health. By providing genetic counselling services, DTC genetic testing companies are drawing on traditional associations of genetic counselling with clinical services and monogenetic testing, associations that carry with them forms of trust. This association includes traditional professional attributes (in this case, those of autonomy, expertise, independence, and non-directedness).

Conclusion

In summary, our analysis suggests the importance of attending not only to the possibilities of 'new' social relations opened when genetics goes online, but to active choices by various actors in how these configurations are played out and represented, particularly when they claim associations with professional qualities that have traditionally engendered trust. Some of these changes represent substantial alterations in social relations, and we argue that such changes are worth noting. For example:

- utilisation of telegenetics for a range of consumers, not only those who are specifically rurally or culturally isolated;
- the genetic counselling profession's entrepreneurial involvement with commercial enterprise; and
- the new kinds of genetic information being provided by GWAS tests, differing from the monogenetic results that genetic counsellors have traditionally dealt with.

Furthermore, changes in scope, temporality and/or spatial organisation of healthcare relations may draw upon associations, such as those of trust, engendered within previous configurations.

The involvement of genetic counsellors and other healthcare professionals in the genetic testing industry also has a role to play in shaping the direct-to-consumer genetic testing product. Not only do genetic counsellors, physicians, and others potentially act as markers of clinical trust on the website, as discussed above, but their presence also raises interesting questions in regard to the 'directness' of genetic tests sold to the consumer, a common point of concern for those critical of DTC genetic testing. As discussed earlier, much research about DTC genetic testing considers 'direct-to-consumer' to mean the selling of genetic tests to the lay public unmediated by a healthcare professional, and this unmediated access is part of the marketing appeal of the product. Our analysis suggests that genetic counsellors introduce a mediating aspect into the service, which has previously been underexplored in the literature, and is relevant to analysis of other healthcare professional involvement. In dealing directly with physicians, either through education or product advice, genetic counsellors working within the DTC genetic testing industry also highlight that we need to consider carefully not only what is meant by 'direct', but also what is meant by 'consumer'.

The DTC genetic testing industry is sometimes portrayed as a service delivery model, a way of getting genetic information into clinical practice, by-passing traditional roles, relationships and forms of expertise and control that structure clinical spaces. We find, as Kenen (1997: 1384) observed in the 1990s, that 'genetic counselors find themselves once again actors in a sociomedical context fraught with ethical and social concerns compounded by changes in the way genetic services are delivered'. The literature is divided between those who argue that genetic counsellors need to be involved with interpretation of DTC genetic testing results, considering their expertise in risk communication and analysis (O'Daniel, 2010; Weaver and Pollin, 2012), and those who argue that DTC genetic testing is outside their jurisdiction, and distracts from 'the real work of answering the questions that counselors have been asked and giving information in which they have real confidence' (Clarke and Thirlaway, 2011).

Rather than take sides in this debate, we have critically explored the roles that genetic counsellors are represented to be assuming as part of the DTC genetic testing industry. Even with regard to this one healthcare profession, our research has raised many questions for further research. For example, normative elements (both represented and manifest in practice) of genetic counselling and DTC genetic testing require closer examination. As Wade and Wilfond (2006: 289) have written, 'simply because a test is "genetic" does not mean that a genetic counsellor is always the clinician best suited to handling the case'. Other genetics experts may be more appropriate in this context, such as genetic nurses (Lea *et al.*, 1998; Weaver and Pollin, 2012), who may be more professionally associated with giving lifestyle advice, as well as having experience with common health conditions. If researchers question the role of telegenetics for 'more complex cases' (Zilliacus *et al.*, 2010: 470), where does this leave the role of telegenetic counselling for complex disease information provided by DTC genetic testing, especially for mental illness which arguably requires greater support (Zilliacus *et al.*, 2010)? If, as Boenink (2008: 60) writes, 'the counseling trajectory can be conceptualized as a shared tinkering with divergent tools and means to fight a host of uncertainties', how will genetic counsellors in the DTC genetic testing industry engage in tinkering with uncertainty through a single phone call or through internet interaction? How will genetic counsellors themselves, as well as other healthcare professionals, use and view the internet, or interactive features of the medium, during their counselling sessions or to otherwise support engagement with patients/consumers? What shifts in the roles and nature of expertise of other healthcare professionals such as physicians, and boundaries among them, are occurring?

In general, little is known about how healthcare professionals in various roles are increasingly becoming entangled with commercial personal genetics as users, producers, mediators, or otherwise, and what they think about what DTC genetic testing means for their profession, their professional identity, and the range of their expertise. How visible (or invisible) are these entanglements? What expectations of action and relationships, and implications for relations of trust, are entailed in these entanglements (trust in professions, trust in institutions such as clinical care and science)? Is there any room left for uncertainty in patient/consumer engagements with healthcare professionals, and how is uncertainty to be recognised and dealt with? How are healthcare professionals dealing with an ambiguous product that absolves itself from diagnosis, is represented on the basis of providing health information, and invites personal, non-clinical tinkering? We also know little about how users are engaging with these genetic counselling services, although recent research has shown a low-uptake of the free genetic counselling offered by one of these sites (Bloss, Schork and Topol, 2011).

Our analysis of one healthcare profession provides an important starting point for further research in this area. We have shown that at least one healthcare profession, genetic counsellors, are represented as assuming shifting roles, with potentially shifting competencies and requirements for expertise as well as ambiguities concerning social relations of trust. The potential diversification of roles for genetic counsellors will help them to maintain a particular position in the healthcare marketplace (Nancarrow and Borthwick, 2005). We argue that, in the examination of social arrangements facilitated by genetics 'going online', our examination of implications for genetic counsellors points toward directions for analysis of other healthcare professions. Crucially, we position these as users of the technology, and take as a starting point the co-production of users and technologies. Second, we point to ambiguity regarding shifts in relationships among actors, such as the spatio-temporal, or nuanced shifts in the deployment of expertise, as having implications for trust relations. We suggest that the visibility or invisibility of these shifts is of importance in the analysis of any healthcare profession.

References

ABGC (2009) *Practice-based competencies*, Lenexa, KS: American Board of Genetic Counseling, available at www.abgc.net/docs/Practice%20Based%20Competencies_ Aug%202006%2010-29-09.pdf (accessed 6 January 2012).

Abrams, D. and Geier, M. (2006) 'A comparison of patient satisfaction with telehealth and on-site consultations: A pilot study for prenatal genetic counseling', *Journal of Genetic Counseling*, vol.15, no. 3, pp. 199–205, doi: 10.1007/s10897-006-9020-0.

American College of Medical Genetics Board of Directors (2004) 'ACMG statement on direct-to-consumer genetic testing', *Genetics in Medicine*, vol. 6, no. 1, p. 60, doi: 10.1097/01.GIM.0000106164.59722.CE.

American Congress of Obstetricians and Gynecologists (2008) 'ACOG committee opinion no. 409: Direct-to-consumer marketing of genetic testing', *Obstetrics and Gynecology*, vol. 111, no. 6, pp. 1493–1494, doi: 10.1097/AOG.0b013e31817d250e.

Arribas-Ayllon, M., Sarangi, S. and Clarke, A. (2012) 'Ethical decision-making in expert and family systems: The dynamics of trust-distrust in genetic testing', paper presented on 29 June at the Tenth Interdisciplinary Conference Communication, Medicine and Ethics, Trondheim, Norway.

Bloss, C. S., Schork, N. J. and Topol, E. J. (2011) 'Effects of direct-to-consumer genomewide profiling to assess disease risk', *New England Journal of Medicine*, vol. 364, no. 6, pp. 524–534.

Boenink, M. (2008) 'Genetic diagnostics for hereditary breast cancer: Displacement of uncertainty and responsibility', in G. de Vries and K. Horstman (eds), *Genetics from laboratory to society*, Basingstoke: Palgrave Macmillan, pp. 37–63.

Clarke, A. and Thirlaway, K. (2011) 'Genomic counseling? Genetic counseling in the genomic era', *Genome Medicine: Medicine in the post genomic era.* vol. 3, no. 1, p. 7, doi:10.1186/gm221.

Couzin, J. (2008) 'Gene tests for psychiatric risk polarize researchers', *Science*, vol. 319, no. 5861, pp. 274–277, doi: 10.1126/science.319.5861.274.

European Society of Human Genetics (2010) 'Statement of the ESHG on direct-to-consumer genetic testing for health-related purposes', *European Journal of Human Genetics*, vol. 18, no. 12,pp. 1271–1273, doi:10.1038/ejhg.2010.129.

Featherstone, K., Atkinson, P., Bharadwaj, A. and Clarke, A. (2006) *Risky relations: Family, kinship and the new genetics*, Oxford: Berg.

Finucane, B. (2012) '2012 National Society of Genetic Counselors Presidential Address: Maintaining our professional identity in an ever-expanding genetics universe', *Journal of Genetic Counseling*, vol. 21, pp. 3–5, doi: 10.1007/s10897-011-9466-6.

Forsythe, D. E. (1996) 'New bottles, old wine: Hidden cultural assumptions in a computerized explanation system for migraine sufferers', *Medical Anthropology Quarterly*, vol. 10, no. 4, pp. 551–574.

Genetics and Public Policy Center (2006) 'Direct-to-consumer genetic testing: empowering or endangering the public?', available at www.dnapolicy.org/policy.issue.php?action=detail&issuebrief_id=32 (accessed 10 May 2011; archived by WebCite at www.webcitation.org/5znzdZmqv).

Genetics and Public Policy Center (2011) 'Direct-to-consumer genetic testing companies', www.dnapolicy.org/news.release.php?action=detail&pressrelease_id=145 (accessed 17 August 2011; archived by WebCite at www.webcitation.org/610DDbCns).

Guttmacher, A. E. and Collins, F. S. (2003) 'Welcome to the genomic era', *New England Journal of Medicine*, vol. 349, no. 10, pp. 996–998, doi:10.1056/NEJMe038132.

Hawkins, A. and Ho, A. (2012) 'Genetic counseling and the ethical issues around direct to consumer genetic testing', *Journal of Genetic Counseling*, vol. 21, no. 3, pp. 367–373, doi: 10.1007/s10897-012-9488-8.

Hennen, L., Sauter, A. and Van Den Cruyce, E. (2010) 'Direct to consumer genetic testing: Insights from an internet scan', *New Genetics and Society*, vol. 29, no. 2, pp. 167–186, doi: 10.1080/14636778.2010.484232.

Hercher, L. (2009) 'DC takes on DTC: The "T" doesn't stand for tomorrow anymore', available at http://thednaexchange.com/2009/09/04/dc-takes-on-dtc-the-t-doesnt-stand-for-tomorrow-anymore (accessed 14 September 2015).

Hock, K., Christensen, K., Yashar, B., Roberts, J. S., Gollust, S. E. and Uhlmann, W. (2011) 'Direct-to-consumer genetic testing: An assessment of genetic counselors' knowledge and beliefs', *Genetics in Medicine*, vol. 13, no. 4, pp. 325–332, doi: 10.1097/GIM.0b013e3182011636.

Howard, H. and Borry, P. (2008) 'Direct-to-consumer genetic testing: More questions than benefits?' Editorial. *Personalised Medicine*, vol. 5, no. 4, pp. 317–320, doi 10.2217/17419541.5.4.31.

Howard, H. and Borry, P. (2012) 'Is there a doctor in the house? The presence of physicians in the direct-to-consumer genetic testing context', *Journal of Community Genetics*, vol. 3, no. 2, pp. 105–112, doi: 10.1007/s12687-011-0062-0.

Hudson, K., Javitt, G., Burke, W., Byers, P. and ASHG Social Issues Committee (2007) 'ASHG statement on direct-to-consumer genetic testing in the United States', *The American Journal of Human Genetics*, vol. 81, pp. 635–637, doi: 10.1097/01.AOG.0000292086.98514.8b.

Jordens, C. F. C., Kerridge, I. H. and Samuel, G. N. (2009) 'Direct-to-consumer personal genome testing: The problem is not ignorance it is market failure', *The American Journal of Bioethics*, vol. 9, no. 6, pp. 13–15, doi: 10.1080/15265160902874411.

Kenen, R. H. (1997) 'Opportunities and impediments for a consolidating and expanding profession: Genetic counseling in the United States', *Social Science and Medicine*, vol. 45, no. 9, pp. 1377–1386, doi: 10.1016/S0277-9536(97)00062-2.

Koch, L. and Nordahl Svendsen, M. (2005) 'Providing solutions-defining problems: The imperative of disease prevention in genetic counselling', *Social Science and Medicine*, vol. 60, no. 4, pp. 823–832, doi: 10.1016/j.socscimed.2004.06.019.

Lea, D. H., Jenkins, J. F. and Francomano, C. A. (1998) *Genetics in clinical practice: New directions for nursing and health care*, Toronto: Jones and Bartlett.

Leighton, J. W., Valverde, K. and Bernhardt, B. A. (2012) 'The general public's understanding and perception of direct-to-consumer genetic test results', *Public Health Genomics*, vol. 15, pp. 11–21, doi: 10.1159/000327159.

McGowan, M. L., Fishman, J. R. and Lambrix, M. A. (2010) 'Personal genomics and individual identities: Motivations and moral imperatives of early users', *New Genetics and Society*, vol. 29, no. 3, pp. 261–290, doi: 10.1080/14636778.2010.507485.

McGowan, M. L., Fishman, J. R., Settersten, R. A. Jr., Lambrix, M. A., Jeungst, E. T. (2014) 'Gatekeepers or intermediaries? The role of clinicians in commercial genomic testing', *PLoS ONE*, vol. 9, no. 9, pp. 1–7, e108484, doi:10.1371/journal.pone.0108484

McGuire, A. L., Diaz, C. M., Wang, T. and Hilsenbeck, S. G. (2009) 'Social networkers' attitudes toward direct-to-consumer personal genome testing', *The American Journal of Bioethics*, vol. 9, no. 6, pp. 3–10, doi: 10.1080/15265160902928209.

Martin, E. (2006) 'Pharmaceutical virtue', *Culture, Medicine and Psychiatry*, vol. 30, no. 2, pp. 157–174, doi: 10.1007/s11013-006-9014-2.

Matloff, E. and Caplan, A. (2008) 'Direct to confusion: Lessons learned from marketing BRCA testing', *The American Journal of Bioethics*, vol. 8, no. 6, pp. 5–8, doi: 10.1080/15265160802248179.

Nancarrow, S. A. and Borthwick, A. M. (2005) 'Dynamic professional boundaries in the healthcare workforce', *Sociology of Health and Illness*, vol. 27, no. 7, pp. 897–919, doi: 10.1111/j.1467-9566.2005.00463.x.

Novas, C. and Rose, N. (2000) 'Genetic risk and the birth of the somatic individual', *Economy and Society*, vol. 29, no. 4, pp. 485–513, doi: 10.1080/03085140050174750.

NSGC (2010a) 'Consumers should be mindful of DTC genetic testing: Don't bypass genetic counselors, medical geneticists or other healthcare providers', available at www.nsgc.org/client_files/news/040609dtc.pdf (accessed 5 May 2011; archived by WebCite at www.webcitation.org/5zx2YwWhX).

NSGC (2010b) 'National Society of Genetic Counselors professional status survey 2010: Executive summary', available at www.nsgc.org/Publications/ProfessionalStatus Survey/tabid/142/Default.aspx (accessed 6 January 2012).

NSGC (2011) 'FAQs about genetic counselors and the NSGC', available at www.nsgc.org/About/FAQsaboutGeneticCounselorsandtheNSGC/tabid/143/Default.as px (accessed 11 August 2012; archived by WebCite at www.webcitation.org/ 60qxjfXLH).

Nuffield Council on Bioethics (2010) *Medical profiling and online medicine: The ethics of 'personalised healthcare' in a consumer age*, London: Nuffield Council on Bioethics.

O'Daniel, J. (2010) 'The prospect of genome-guided preventive medicine: A need and opportunity for genetic counselors', *Journal of Genetic Counseling*, vol. 19, no. 4, pp. 315–327, doi: 10.1007/s10897-010-9302-4.

Oldani, M. J. (2004) 'Thick prescriptions: Toward an interpretation of pharmaceutical sales practices', *Medical Anthropology Quarterly*, vol. 18, no. 3, pp. 325–356, doi: 10.1525/maq.2004.18.3.325.

Pagon, R. A. (2002) 'Genetic testing for disease susceptibilities: Consequences for genetic counseling', *Trends in Molecular Medicine*, vol. 8, no. 6, pp. 306–307, doi: 10.1016/S1471-4914(02)02348-1.

Petrakaki, D., Cornford, T., Hibberd, R., Lichtner, V. and Barber, N. (2011) 'The role of technology in shaping the professional future of community pharmacists: The case of the electronic prescription service in the English National Health Service', *Researching the Future in Information Systems*, vol. 356, pp. 179–195, doi: 10.1007/978-3-642-21364-9_12.

Powell, K., Christianson, C., Cogswell, W., Dave, G., Verma, A., Eubanks, S. and Henrich, V. (2012) 'Educational needs of primary care physicians regarding direct-to-consumer genetic testing', *Journal of Genetic Counseling*, vol. 21, no. 3, pp. 469–478, doi: 10.1007/s10897-011-9471-9.

Prosser, H. and Walley, T. 2006, 'New drug prescribing by hospital doctors: The nature and meaning of knowledge', *Social Science and Medicine*, vol. 62, no. 7, pp. 1565–1578, doi: 10.1016/j.socscimed.2005.08.035.

Rees, G., Young, M.-A., Gaff, C. and Martin, P. (2006) 'A qualitative study of health professionals' views regarding provision of information about health-protective behaviors during genetic consultation for breast cancer', *Journal of Genetic Counseling*, vol. 15, no. 2, pp. 95–104, doi: 10.1007/s10897-005-9009-0.

Richards, M. (2010) 'Reading the runes of my genome: A personal exploration of retail genetics', *New Genetics and Society*, vol. 29, no. 3, pp. 291–310, doi: 10.1080/14636778.2010.507486.

Skirton, H., Lewis, C., Kent, A. and Coviello, D. A. (2010) 'Genetic medicine and the challenge of genomic medicine: Development of core competencies to support preparation of health professionals in Europe', *European Journal of Human Genetics*, vol. 18, pp. 972–977, doi: 10.1038/ejhg.2010.64.

Stalker, H. J., Wilson, R., McCune, H., Gonzalez, J, Moffett, M. and Zori, R. T. (2006) 'Telegenetic medicine: improved access to services in an underserved area', *Journal of Telemedicine and Telecare*, vol. 12, no. 4, pp. 182–185, doi: 10.1258/ 135763306777488762.

Udesky, L. (2010) 'The ethics of direct-to-consumer genetic testing', *The Lancet*, vol. 376, no. 9750, pp. 1377–1378, doi:10.1016/S0140-6736(10)61939-3.

Wade, C. H. and Wilfond, B. S. (2006) 'Ethical and clinical practice considerations for genetic counselors related to direct-to-consumer marketing of genetic tests', *American*

Journal of Medical Genetics Part C: Seminars in Medical Genetics, vol. 142C, no. 4, pp. 284–292, doi: 10.1002/ajmg.c.30110.

Waltho, S. (2011) 'Learning to create opportunity', available at http://thednaexchange.com/2011/03/17/learning-to-create-opportunity (accessed 15 September 2015).

Weaver, M. and Pollin, T. (2012) 'Direct-to-consumer genetic testing: What are we talking about?', *Journal of Genetic Counseling*, vol. 21, no. 3, pp. 361–366, doi: 10.1007/s10897-012-9493-y.

Williams-Jones, B. and Graham, J. E. (2003) 'Actor-network theory: A tool to support ethical analysis of commercial genetic testing', *New Genetics and Society*, vol. 22, no. 3, pp. 271–296, doi: 10.1080/1463677032000147225.

Wyatt, S., Harris, A., Adams, S. and Kelly, S. (2013) 'Illness online: Self-reported data and questions of trust in medical and social research', *Theory, Culture and Society*, vol. 30, no. 4, pp. 131–150.

Zilliacus, E., Meiser, B., Lobb, E., Kirk, J., Warwick, L. and Tucker, K. (2010) 'Women's experience of telehealth cancer genetic counseling', *Journal of Genetic Counseling*, vol. 19, no. 5, pp. 463–472, doi: 10.1007/s10897-010-9301-5.

4   Participation

At the beginning of the first chapter, you made your entry into genetic testing. You sent your money and your saliva to a genetic testing company, and received your results. Perhaps, like some of the testers in the YouTube videos we looked at in Chapter 2, you tried to make sense of the data that purports to tell you about your genetic ancestry or your chances of getting a range of diseases. You might think that you have paid for a service, received the information, and that is the end of your relationship with the company. But there is more. Next time you log into your account, a pop-up box appears. You answer some simple questions. Surveys such as 'Ten things about you', 'Health habits' and 'Ten more things about you' appear regularly in your account. These surveys are enticing and fun, even slightly addictive. The company lets you know that its consent form has changed, and gives you an opportunity to click to sign the new form, which you will not see again unless you look for it. You are now cordially being invited to participate in a research 'revolution' ('Please help us to personalise and improve healthcare by contributing to meaningful discoveries made through genetic research!'), giving the company the right to use your genetic data and survey information, but with assurances that your privacy will be protected as much as possible (and your contact and payment information will not be shared).

People who enter the DTC genetic testing marketplace and provide a saliva sample (or cheek swab or blood sample) not only learn about their own genetic information, but also receive invitations to engage in various participatory practices. Companies such as 23andMe invite its customers to share genetic information with other users, to find 'relatives', to post comments on community fora and to become involved in research. In this chapter, we focus on this last form of participation. Not only do individuals send a sample of their saliva, if they engage in the various surveys and other activities as described above they continue to provide data and information. Information is returned to customers in the form of raw genetic test results, analysis and interpretation of genetic data, plus additional material on the company website, blogs and fora about genetics, genetic testing and other company activities. Information is also shared between users, as they can openly invite or search for others to view their genetic results, and through the user-generated content on various 23andMe platforms. In this chapter, we raise the question of why so many people have given, and continue to give, online genetic testing so much information and whether this constitutes participation or some other relationship.

Individuals are increasingly being invited into participatory medical practices, to be 'patients 2.0'. DTC genetic testing is at the forefront of this development, and it is often promoted as participatory medicine *par excellence*. Participation refers not only to buying genetic tests online, but also to other forms of 'participatory' practices into which consumers are enticed once they enter the marketplace, such as sharing genetic profiles, commenting on fora and blogs and taking part in genetic research. In this chapter we examine how consumers of genetic testing companies were enrolled into the research activities of the companies, in particular, 23andMe. 23andMe has promoted what they consider to be a revolutionary model for genetic research, one that collects genetic, health and other information from their customers, via its website. We examine this so-called novel direction in medical research through online self-reporting, as a form of participation. We consider how these participation practices, technologies and markets are intertwined, and their paradoxical potential to be both alienating and emancipatory, to promote personalised healthcare by sharing data with large data bases while trusting that individual privacy was and will continue to be protected. In critically examining the broader cultural processes at work we focus on the economic underpinnings of online participation and the free labour of participants. This chapter looks at what it means to self-report data and the issues of trust that are enmeshed in these models of research which promise to have an impact on how data collection, research participation and biomedical research more broadly are considered.

How does a company that encourages self-reporting by individuals represent and establish trust in its products, services, and data sharing procedures, and in its means for interacting not only with its customers but also with its investors and research partners? We address this question through our focus on a company that uses genetic and phenotypic data provided by their customers to conduct research. We begin with a short review of the developing relationship between the 'participatory turn' in medicine and the role of reporting data through technology. We then outline the research methods utilised by 23andMe which the company celebrated as participatory, as part of a gift exchange. We discuss how this entailed implications of reciprocal ties and was established on free labour.

The participatory turn?

Genetic testing sold through the internet has captured the interest of researchers in various disciplines, including ethics, law and sociology. In such literature, the focus is on the privacy of participants, the representativeness of research cohorts, and the reliability of self-reported data (Hall and Gartner, 2009: 54; Levina, 2010: 6). 23andMe has attempted to address all of these concerns in various ways, with statements in their terms of service, blog posts and research articles about security, privacy and transparency (Do *et al.*, 2011), as well as in their evolving consent documents. These issues are all important, but there are other aspects of 23andMe's research agenda which deserve attention; issues which 23andMe has not addressed, and which are at the very core of their business practice. Richard Tutton and Barbara Prainsack have introduced some of these broader social and economic issues in their study of what they term a 'participatory turn' in disease research (Prainsack, 2011; Tutton and Prainsack, 2011). Their work compares DTC genetic testing research practices to those of population biobanks, examining the 'entrepreneurial' subjectivities of DTC genetic testing participants. We address participation in personal genomics research not only in relation to conventional medical research, but also in the context of web 2.0 practices, an area which Tutton and Prainsack touch upon only briefly.

There may be a 'participatory turn' occurring in the context of DTC genetic testing, but patients, citizens and 'experience-based experts' (Collins and Evans, 2002) have been participating in scientific and medical research endeavours for centuries (e.g. Star and Griesemer, 1989; Lawrence, 2006; McCray, 2006). The participation of patient advocacy groups has been discussed in relation to myopathies (Callon and Rabeharisoa, 2003, 2008), human immunodeficiency virus (Epstein, 2008), stem cell research (Langstrup, 2011), autism and Tourette syndrome (Panofsky, 2011). What differs in the 23andMe context is not only the kinds of agency attributed to research participants, but most importantly for this chapter, the digital dimension of participation, where online platforms, large datasets and computational abilities allow new kinds of participation in research. Within the healthcare context, broadly defined, online participation covers a variety of practices, including the counterparts to those mentioned above, such as online patient advocacy (Akrich, 2010), sharing of patient experiences (Adams, 2010), as well as newer forms of participation facilitated by social media such as health hacking and providing data for medical research. Our contribution to the citizen science/participatory patient literature is, as discussed in Chapter 1, to bring together our understanding of DTC genetic testing with those internet practices which promise to affect how data collection, research participation, and medical research more broadly are considered.

In this chapter we draw upon and bring together internet studies scholarship concerning participatory culture, and sociological literature concerning medical research participation. These literatures deal with remarkably similar themes such as gift exchange, empowerment, democratisation of information and free labour. We utilise four theoretical concepts: gift exchange (Mauss, 1970), free labour (Terranova, 2000), clinical labour (Mitchell and Waldby, 2010), and trust (Shapin and Schaffer, 1985) that illuminate important aspects of online research participation. Gift exchange concerns reciprocity and sociality, whereas free labour and clinical labour concern the provision of services (data entry or physical work) in order to generate economic value. By combining these insights with an analysis of a wide array of web material (see Appendix A for details of methods and materials analysed, and for our reflection on our own position as researchers in the online environment of user-generated data), we offer unique insights into the emerging area of online genetic research.

Novel methods: the 'research-y' part of 23andMe

> I'm more interested in the research-y aspects of it. The fact that you guys have started actually asking questions and relating that to ongoing research I think is interesting. That direction is interesting. It just seems like it's a great repository of information.
>
> (John G, customer testimonial posted by 23andMe on its website)

With significant fanfare and much champagne at one of their famous spit parties, 23andMe was launched in 2007 by Linda Avey and Anne Wojcicki (see Chapter 1). From the outset, the duo made it clear that with this company they wanted to develop research capacity and make a significant contribution to genetic research. A strong advocate for this approach was Wojcicki's then-husband (when the company started), and co-founder of Google, Sergey Brin. With his genetically inherited 'algorithmic sensibility' (Goetz, 2010), *Wired* magazine suggests that this is the man who wants to 'bypass centuries of epistemology in favour of a more Googley kind of science' (Goetz, 2010). These internet research pioneers had an explicit goal not only in replicating and contributing to medical research, but most importantly, in 'revolutionising' research. 23andMe wanted to build 'an entirely new model for conducting research' and 'set the standard for web-based genetic studies' (Eriksson *et al.*, 2010: 17). Avey and Wojcicki saw an opportunity to combine what they saw as an enthusiasm for participation on the internet with cheap genetic analysis, in order to create what they hoped would become one of the world's largest research projects. To this end, 23andMe unveiled its research arm, 23andWe, in May 2008.

23andWe is based on what the company describes as 'participant-led', 'patient-driven', 'consumer-enabled', or 'customer-driven' research methodologies (Eriksson *et al.*, 2010; Do *et al.*, 2011). These methods utilised a combination of consumers' genetic information, analysed from saliva samples, and their phenotype data, obtained via these same people completing online surveys on the 23andMe website. By mid-2011, 23andMe were reporting that more than three-quarters of its 100,000 customers had agreed to take part in research activities, with 60 per cent having taken surveys and hundreds submitting research topics. At the time of our research, 23andMe had published three research articles based on these data: two genome-wide association studies (GWAS) (one for Parkinson's disease and another for common traits such as freckling, ability to smell asparagus in your urine, and sneezing in sunlight), and a study that replicated 180 known genetic associations for medically-related conditions. Each article was authored by company researchers and associates. The company also relied on so-called traditional science articles in order to justify their choice of genetic markers for analysis. An important aspect of these publications was the celebration and validation of web-based methodologies: the authors emphasised not only how their research shows replication and novel genetic associations but also that online self-reported data was a 'viable alternative to traditional methods' (Eriksson *et al.*, 2010: 2).

23andMe claimed that its 'novel study design' (Do *et al.*, 2011) was different from existing research models in three ways. First, 23andMe claimed that its research process was fast. Slow research was seen to 'hamper' progress (Tung *et al.*, 2011), whereas computational techniques allow fast analysis of large data sets, implicitly assumed to improve the nature of scientific research. The 23andMe approach meant efficient recruitment and time saved on collecting information from medical records, the common data source for more 'traditional' studies.

Second, 23andMe claimed novelty through its ability to generate significant numbers of research participants. For 23andMe, large numbers outweighed any errors that may have arisen from self-reported data. Large population samples are needed to attain statistical power in genetic research, especially in GWAS which detect subtle genetic effects. GWAS are reliant upon and stimulating advances in information technologies that enable large data storing capacity. Substantial databases were created by 23andMe using what many genetic researchers would disregard: incomplete data or partially completed surveys; in their published papers self-reported data of varying degrees of completeness were used. 23andMe's cohort was also unique in that it was continually expanding, with participants participating in multiple studies in parallel. Because new participants were joining the studies at all times, the results were also continuously changing (Eriksson *et al.*, 2010: 15).

Third, 23andMe (2008) claimed that their research approach differed from traditional research because it was completely 'web-based'. This claim ignores the many material practices involved, such as spitting and processing spit, and the lab work undertaken to analyse samples; nonetheless the web-based methods are highlighted as a novel feature:

> We're at the beginning of a revolution that combines genetics and the Internet. Wikipedia, YouTube and MySpace have all changed the world by empowering individuals to share information. We believe this same phenomenon can revolutionize healthcare.

The methods used by 23andMe do not rely on collecting information from paper records, and individuals from around the world can take part. 23andMe used the internet to recruit research participants from its customer base via blog posts, tweets, forum posts and announcements on its website, as well as through a pop-up window when returning customers log-in. This approach was claimed to alleviate the difficulties faced by more traditional medical researchers in identifying and recruiting participants (Williams *et al.*, 2008: 1451; Allison, 2009: 895; Terry and Terry, 2011: 1), particularly participants who do not live near research centres; accumulating large enough data sets; and conducting costly and time-intensive research. We now turn to examine how these web-based research methods tie into the 'participatory culture' of 23andMe.

23andMe's 'participatory culture'

Those surveys we mentioned in the introduction to this chapter looked remarkably similar to the easy-to-answer surveys collecting consumer buying behaviour information in order to make personalised product recommendations. Rather than your favourite board game or holiday destination, 23andMe survey questions were about pulse rates, cholesterol levels, eye colour and family history, or they might simply have asked, 'Have you ever been diagnosed by a doctor with [Condition X]'? 23andMe survey designers wanted to keep participation high by having only easy and quick tasks (Tung *et al.*, 2011) that make 'the survey-taking experience simpler, more interesting, and more rewarding' (23andMe, 2009). This contributed to the pleasurable and recreational aspects of research participation. Involvement in some surveys was more elaborate, such as the Parkinson's Disease survey which involves participants filling in a general medical questionnaire, contributing information about disease progression, other diagnoses, symptoms and response to medication (Do *et al.*, 2011).

Participation was kept flexible – 'participate in research at your own pace. Answer a few questions or answer them all' – but it was always encouraged – 'the more active you are in the community, the more you'll get out of it' (23andMe, 2011a). 23andMe acknowledged that only limited information can be obtained from the simple questions that most consumer-participants answer in the brief surveys, and that more information may need to be obtained by going back to the cohort to ask more in-depth questions, and potentially even conduct in-person visits (Tung *et al.*, 2011).

23andMe customers also 'participated' in research activities more implicitly. Various kinds of data were used by the company. Genetic data and self-reported data of those customers who provided informed consent were used explicitly in research, as described above, but also the genetic data of all customers, regardless of consent, were used in aggregated sets for internal validation experiments, and to develop new features and products. User-generated content such as feedback on fora and blog comments fed into the company's research design. Users' web activity was also collected through log files, cookies and web beacon technology, so that web behaviour data, including our own as social science researchers, were used by 23andMe (2011b) in order to monitor use of its website, to improve its services and to tailor and customise content for customers.

The participatory potential inherent in these research activities was indeed questionable. Participation in research essentially consisted of 'allowing 23andMe investigators to access your Genetic & Self-Reported Information' (23andMe, 2015) A funding statement made in a 23andMe research article highlighted this: 'the study was funded by the participants, by 23andMe, and a grant from Sergey Brin [Google] ... The funders had no role in the study design, data collection and analysis, decision to publish, or preparation of the manuscript' (Do *et al.*, 2011). Dolgin (2010: 954) argues that while 23andMe's *PLoS* paper 'bolstered the notion of decentralised, participant-driven research, all of the contributors remained relatively passive, doing little more than responding to a questionnaire and signing an informed consent form to share their data'. Ultimately, the company controlled all forms of participation on the website, as outlined in the terms of service, rules for engagement on forums and in the 23andMe (2011c) research design whereby the company 'enabled' consumers to participate.

The participatory culture of 23andMe research thus appears considerably different to disease-specific patient-organised research participation. We do not see the symmetrical forms of expertise which Callon and Rabeharisoa (2003) argue are created in a trading zone of circulating genetic and experiential information among patient advocacy organisations and professional researchers. Neither do we get a sense of the transformative potential for patients (Epstein, 2008; Panofsky, 2011: 32), nor the emotional investment of patients and affected families hoping to advance diagnosis and treatment of their illness. Our purpose here is not to judge the extent of participation, but rather to look at how the research was *represented* on the website, and what kind of participatory practices emerged as a result. We focus particularly on how 23andMe represents research participation as a form of sociality, facilitated through gift exchange.

Sharing gifts under the genetic family tree

Through participation in this genetic research, and on the internet more broadly, new forms of network sociality were enacted between known and previously unknown individuals. Internet scholars have approached the sociality of participation in various ways. For some time, literature was divided between celebratory and culturally pessimistic viewpoints on the forms of social life being promoted, created and resisted on the web (Rheingold, 2002; Surowiecki, 2004; Jenkins, 2006; Karaganis, 2007; Bruns, 2008). There are more nuanced accounts, focusing on how participation practices, technology, markets and politics are intertwined (Schäfer, 2011) and paradoxical in terms of their potential to be both alienating and emancipatory (Proulx *et al.*, 2011). Some scholars highlight the economic underpinnings of online participation (Terranova, 2000; Goldberg, 2011; Proulx *et al.*, 2011; Jordan, 2015), and critically examine the broader cultural processes at work. We align ourselves with these more critical approaches towards participatory cultures. We acknowledge that involvement in 23andMe research may be rewarding for the consumer–participant, but it is also financially rewarding for the company. While consumer and company may both be driven by an individualistic consumer culture, ultimately 23andMe accumulated the greatest (financial) benefit.

It is unsurprising therefore that 23andMe celebrated what it promoted as the emancipatory aspects of participating in the genetic research revolution. Enthusiastic statements made by participants were posted on the website, tweeted and retweeted. 23andMe claimed to provide a platform for users to have a voice and to have greater input in genetic research. In doing so, the company drew upon two complementary discourses concerning the democratising and empowering potential of the internet and of personal genomics as described in Chapter 1.

Within this celebratory context, 23andMe promoted research participation as a form of gift-exchange. In signing the consent form, customers relinquished all rights to any financial gain from research; instead gifts were represented as being exchanged, via the internet. People first offered their money and their spit, swimming with cheek cells which hold the all-important DNA. This occurred initially as a commercial exchange, whereby the 23andMe laboratories analysed the genetic contents of the drool, and returned the results back to the paying customer. The remainder of the spit was discarded but the genetic information became part of a database. Customers were then offered the chance to be involved in research. This was when the meaning ascribed to the sample, or the genetic information derived from it (Tutton, 2002: 537), became a 'gift', from the paying customer to 23andMe researchers.

This relationship appeared to be alien to the 'potential users or non-users' we interviewed. Several commented that the company should be paying them to use their DNA other than the other way around. Typically, one respondent said: 'That's the thing, you know if they want to see my genetics … 'cause they're going to make a business out of it, not me. They should be paying me to see my genetics.' Another commented: 'Mmm, so they take out the DNA and hold onto that? They haven't bought it from you, have they?'

This gift, however, held little value in itself. The power of GWAS is in large quantities of data, data which are a combination of genotypic and phenotypic information. 23andMe not only needed lots of DNA, but it needed to link this to consumers' personal information about their pulse rates, olfactory skills and neurological symptoms. This is where individuals were represented as engaging in further aspects of gift exchange, by providing personal information via the completion of surveys. As sharing this information took time and effort, no matter how simple the questions were, 23andMe needed to give gifts in return, as incentives for participation (Eysenbach, 2008: 6). These gifts were presented as returned results, acknowledgement and badges.

In much of the 23andMe web material, there was an emphasis on feeding research results back to participants:

> We believe research is a two-way process, where participants are valued as partners in scientific discovery. As part of our commitment to involving everyone in the research process, we've launched 23andMe Research Findings [hyperlink], a regularly updated public gallery of some of the latest findings to come out of our ongoing research … we still feel it's important to keep everyone updated on our progress, especially those who have contributed to the research effort.
>
> (23andMe, 2011d)

23andMe used various platforms in order to share results with its users and participants, such as forum comments, 'research snippets' on the website, tweets and blog posts. Results were fed back to participants throughout the research process, from immediately after completing the surveys, when participants can see how they compared to others, to blog posts about recently published research articles, to research updates and snippets of information on consumer care websites.

Participants also received the gift of acknowledgement in these publications, being thanked for participating 'enthusiastically' (Do *et al.*, 2011), despite control exercised by the company, articulated in the consent forms as outlined above.

Embroidered onto the virtual lapels of research participants' profiles were badges of participation. These badges appeared as green or blue dots near users' avatars, denoting them as 'research pioneers' or 'research trailblazers'. Like the badges offered to users for voting or posting comments on the user-generated online TV network Current TV (Fish *et al.*, 2011: 31), these icons were used as symbols and rewards of activity valued by the company, encouraging further participation. 23andMe users were socialised into their cultural value, these gifts being visible signs to others of participation, their social value confirmed through recognition and reputation (Proulx *et al.*, 2011: 13). 23andMe consumer-partici-pants also became 'research captains' by recruiting other participants to form a research community. Captains supposedly had the opportunity to 'speak to the research team about what research is done and how' (Allison, 2009: 898), although their actual involvement in research conducted by 23andMe was unclear. Nonetheless, these discourses show that participation was rewarded, and the active, perpetually engaged, responsible citizen-consumer promoted (Adams, 2010: 192; Tutton and Prainsack, 2011: 4).

23andMe used a variety of internet platforms in combination, taking advantage, in its words, of the 'interactivity' of the web (Eriksson *et al.*, 2010), not only to recruit participants, but also to accept and return what were offered as gifts. Digital gift exchange has long been a topic of interest in internet studies (Bergquist and Ljungberg, 2001; Pearson, 2007), particularly through the work of Barbrook (2005) who argues that gift exchange and market exchange not only co-exist but are symbiotic, in what he describes as a 'mixed economy'. In medical sociology, the notion of gift exchange has also been used to understand donation of bodily matter such as blood (Tutton, 2002), semen (Tober, 2001), stem cells (Waldby, 2002) and organs (Shaw, 2012). Many of these researchers recognise that human tissue can pass through various spheres of exchange, becoming a gift at one moment and a commodity at another (Lipworth *et al.*, 2011: 805), the distinction between the two blurring (Tober, 2001: 140). In the case of spitting for 23andMe, the human material was not 'donated', but rather began as part of a commercial exchange in which the customer paid the company to analyse the material. It was 23andMe who then attempted to blur the material into part of a gift exchange.

This bears similarity to the kinds of 'economies' identified in other practices around donated tissue that gains value when circulating into the hands and agen-das of a different range of actors. For example, drawing from literature on the bio-economy (e.g. Mitchell and Waldby, 2010), Julie Kent (2008) has reported on the exchange relationship among women undergoing abortion, clinicians, and stem cell scientists in Britain. She identifies that important in the relationships within which tissues circulate are variable consent procedures and procurement practices.

Biomedical research, much social science, and user-generated content online all rely on individuals contributing material without financial remuneration. While some participants may receive more tangible benefits from participation, such as access to drugs or payment for their online contributions, for most contributors to both medical research and other online forms of contribution, participation incurs intangible benefits such as enhanced self-worth, enhanced reputation, a sense of contributing to the public good, personal satisfaction, and the prospect of future reward or reciprocity (Tutton, 2002: 526; Pearson, 2007; Williams *et al.*, 2008: 1452; Hallowell *et al.*, 2010; Li, 2011; Lipworth *et al.*, 2011). In the next section, we focus on one particular aspect of gift exchange, the obligations of reciprocity.

Reciprocal ties

According to the anthropologist Marcel Mauss (1970), gift giving always entails reciprocal exchange and hidden ties of mutual obligation. The consumer can be read to have an implicit obligation to participate, to give gifts and to accept them in return, this being part and parcel of the economic exchange. This reciprocal exchange ties people together creating 'social interdependencies' (Bergquist and Ljungberg, 2001: 308). In her study of the social media platform LiveJournal, Pearson (2007) writes that gift exchange is part of social practice that acts to 'bond together participants, making the individuals feel connected and linked into something larger than their own immediate social (internodal) connections'. In this vein, our analysis suggests that 23andMe used gift exchange as a way of trying to create social bonds with customers. According to social psychologists, stronger integrative bonds are formed when reciprocity is constant (Molm, 2010: 125). 23andMe continuously offered gifts to its customers, to facilitate participation, and create stronger social ties to its research agenda.

In order to facilitate these social bonds, 23andMe fostered the development of communities, attempting to establish *communitas* (Turner 1969), perhaps even attempting to replicate the patient group models which have become so active in research. In their community guidelines, 23andMe (2011a) stated, 'Write. Your contributions strengthen the community … Share. We want to provide you the opportunity to connect to and create communities around common interests, affinities and passions.' Users were encouraged on various platforms to build research groups and comment on fora, as well as share genetic data with others. Sharing formed the basis of these communal and social bonds, and the framework for the research methodology, a constructed attempt at bio-sociality.

While 23andMe promoted a sociable gift exchange within its formulated feel-good atmosphere (Prainsack, 2011: 139), we argue that these bonds were ultimately created in order to build a large, unique, and profitable database. Rather than a web of warm and fuzzy social connections, what 23andMe wanted was a loyal, 're-contactable cohort':

A platform like this one that maintains an ongoing relationship with the participants, including sharing data with them, may motivate individuals to participate and stay active in research … As we move into studies that require ever larger sample sizes … making optimal use of our resources will become a necessity. We believe that this model in which investigators maintain long-term relationships with research participants and facilitate their participation through online tools is a significant step in that direction.

(Tung *et al.*, 2011: 10)

The social ties created by 23andMe were superficial or weak ties (Granovetter, 1973), implying a form of pseudo-regard rather than relations of regard (Offer, 1997), in which sociality was established for the economic advantage of the company. A large 'recontactable cohort' is a valuable resource for researchers wanting to perform longitudinal genetic research, particularly epigenetic research. In 2011, 23andMe (2011e) offered free tests to 100,000 potential customers of African descent, suggesting they needed to create incentives in order to create a more representative database of racially diverse research participants, a resource which is showing, in the long run, to be a greater revenue generator than the genetic tests themselves, considering the sale of the databases recently to Genetech (Saxena, 2015).

The inconsistent language used to refer to participants reflects how the 23andMe business agenda was not made completely visible to consumers. On the 23andMe website encouraging participation, users were referred to as collaborators, advisers and contributors, whereas in research articles 23andMe stated that they can 'improve replication success by taking advantage of our recontactable cohort' (Tung *et al.*, 2011). In a TEDMED presentation, those who participated online were referred to by Anne Wojcicki as 'active genomes'.

Social ties created through participation form a network, which expands. Sharing becomes good for the network, for the company (Levina, 2010: 5). Communities become hollow in this light, the word arguably losing strength more broadly in the context of online cultural production (Schäfer, 2011: 17). Collectivity emerges then independent of a sense of community (Proulx *et al.*, 2011: 17). By providing resources for the research agenda of the company, the collective fuels profits, becoming a form of free labour.

Enticements to provide free labour, and data, largely though additional consumption, are an interesting element of the continuing relationship 23andMe sought to maintain with its customers (the intersection of consumption and free labour is one to which we want to call attention, facilitated as it is by 'digital relations' including advertising and complex algorithms that track and predict consumer's preferences). For example, 23andMe has advertised to existing customers suggestions of buying additional tests for relatives on occasions such as Mother's Day. Along with other forms of 'play' and the pleasure of consumption, the company makes much of the 'power' of genetics to find (and form and inform) families, while at the same time gaining access to familial lineages. Participation, like community, takes on a different, thinner meaning, when the nature of participation is less than transparent.

Participating in medical research in the context of this mixture of relationships of different natures was viewed with some scepticism by the respondents we interviewed. One respondent described her perspective as follows:

Oh, mmm, participating in research, yes, for a commercial enterprise, probably not if, if the ultimate gain was going to be increased dividends for shareholders. That would not be a good enough reason, if the ultimate goal is going to be improved understanding and genuine empowerment, possibly. So if … if there was an academic research project looking at the link between my circumstances, the pineal function and depression or hormone levels and depression, I'd be very interested in that … and that might improve a lot of people subsequently, but those might be quite narrow, specific interests.

Spitting for free

The gift exchange promoted by 23andMe created social ties for the benefit of a research network, which we argue, following Tiziana Terranova (2000), was based on free labour. Terranova argues that the various participatory activities of online users are in fact forms of free labour which are structural to late capitalist cultural economy. She writes that 'especially since 1994, the Internet is always and simultaneously a gift economy *and* an advanced capitalist economy. The mistake of the neoliberals (as exemplified by the *Wired* group), is to mistake this coexistence for a benign, unproblematic equivalence' (Terranova, 2000: 51). The problematic nature of the economic underpinnings of online participation has been taken up by other scholars (Goldberg, 2011; Proulx *et al.*, 2011) who, using a variety of empirical examples, further highlight how online contribution participates in the creation of economic value, forming the invisible labour force supporting informational capitalism (Proulx *et al.*, 2011: 9). As Serge Proulx and colleagues (2011: 10) write, 'the giants of the Internet industry are building their industrial and commercial empires through the aggregation of data supplied voluntarily and freely by Internet users'.

The kinds of free labour which 23andMe users undertook included spitting, posting (both packages and forum comments), logging in, filling in surveys and answering other more trivial looking questions, and forming (research, relatedness) communities. Consumer-participants also maintained their internet connections, hardware and software and visited the 23andMe website. 23andMe relied upon all of these activities to perform research. The genetic testing company did not recognise consumer practices as labour, free or otherwise, or as 'value', instead it highlighted the ease and simplicity of participation, stating that self-reporting was done with little effort:

> Traditional methods of data collection – for example, using an existing medical record or a meeting between a researcher and each participant – can be costly, time-consuming and limit the number of people willing and able to participate. In contrast, 23andMe utilizes simple online surveys that can be completed anywhere at anytime. This allows people from all over the world to easily participate in our research on an on-going basis.
>
> (23andMe, 2010)

23andMe did perform some work of its own, by analysing the spit, or by arranging for its laboratory scientists at the National Genetics Institute to do so. It also stored the genetic information, provided tools and a platform for consumers to access their raw data, and created fora for consumers to exchange information. 23andMe (2011f) wrote that its recipe for research was to 'give people tools, add passion, and shake'. The work done by 23andMe, however, was done to add biovalue (Mitchell and Waldby, 2010: 336), by reformulating living matter and living processes into matters of intellectual property and sources of profit (Waldby, 2002: 310). Pálsson (2009a, 2009b) has previously identified these 'biosocial relations of production', commenting on how spitting work contributes to global networks and hierarchies involved in the manufacture of biovalue.

Participation in 23andMe research had similarities to other forms of online free labour. Participants performed simple tasks for rewards, while the companies benefited from the aggregated data. In a very literal Maussian sense of the gift, 23andMe customers gave something of themselves through their engagement with the company's participatory culture. While contributing this bodily material may have initially taken place within the context of a commercial transaction, 23andMe transformed the sample into a gift for their research database. The consumer/participant not only performed free labour, but also performed clinical labour by spitting into the spittoon and submitting it for analysis, the heart of 23andMe's research endeavour.

Mitchell and Waldby (2010: 334) define clinical labour as a form of embodied biomedical work that produces economic value. Clinical labour describes how individuals give clinics and commercial biomedical institutions access to their *in vitro* biology (Mitchell and Waldby, 2010: 339), which is used as a primary resource. New forms of clinical labour are emerging, such as the contribution of genetic material, tissue samples and stem cells to biobanks. Contributing bodily material, whether it is semen, spit or stem cells, is not only a physical act but also a symbolic gesture imbued with cultural value. While some forms of clinical labour are more onerous than spitting, such as submitting your body to daily tests as a 'live-in guinea pig' (Abadie, 2010), thinking about spitting as a form of clinical labour nonetheless helps to understand the economic dimensions underlying consumer/participants' activities.

Genetic information isolated from a saliva sample remains linked to the individual from which it derives, and further health information can therefore be linked to these specimens (Mitchell and Waldby, 2010: 346). Through the aggregated forms of clinical and online free labour performed by thousands of customers, 23andMe has created a research resource with significant economic potential (Mitchell and Waldby, 2010: 348; Saxena, 2015). Following from Pálsson (2009a), in many ways the participant can be seen to be taking part in the *coproduction* of biovalue, for the benefit of the company, rather than in more symmetrical forms of coproduction of scientific knowledge evident in some studies of patient advocacy group involvement in research (see for example Rabeharisoa, Moriera and Akrich, 2014). In different forms of relationship, including economic but also including membership defining, rule-setting, and rhetorical enrolment, users are co-produced in different ways. 23andMe did not completely hide its economic intentions, but nor did it actively promote them. This is a form of pseudo-transparency, where actions are made towards disclosure and transparency but in such a way as to require more than usual diligence on the part of all participants to identify the nature of relationships involved. (Pseudo-transparency on the part of 23andMe was identified via the autoethnographic engagement of Kelly with 23andMe testing, as discussed in Chapter 1 and Appendix A, although it may describe that engagement as well. At the least, the concept suggests critical appraisal of claims regarding the nature of relationships involved in transactions, and research.) Statements about commercial gain can be found in the privacy statement, which stated that '23andMe may enter into commercial arrangements to enable partners to provide our service to their customers and/or to provide you access to their products and services. We may collect fees for these referrals' (23andMe, 2011b).

In this statement, 23andMe acknowledged that it had a resource which gave it significant pharmaceutical (Prainsack and Wolinsky, 2010) and diagnostic biocapital (Mitchell and Waldby, 2010: 337). Data could be sold to any third party who was interested and with whom 23andMe wished to enter into a commercial exchange. Since our empirical data collection, 23andMe has sold its database to the biotechnology firm Genentech, and it has applied for patents regarding gene sharing, novel polymorphisms associated with Parkinson's disease. As a commercial business, 23andMe has a responsibility to provide a return to its numerous investors, who invested more than US$31 million in the first five years of the company's existence. A transaction that began as a commercial exchange ended in commercial exchange, and participation was turned into private profit.

It seems therefore that there was a focus not only on profits obtained from the sale of genetic tests, but also the potential of the research database to generate revenue from pharmaceutical companies, other biotechnology firms, and through the development of patents. In order to secure these profits however, the company potentially jeopardised its trust relations with consumers, as highlighted when the company announced its first novel genetic association patent on their blog. While there were several positive comments about this development, the reaction from consumers was largely hostile, many considering that they had been 'duped' into participating into this revenue-generating venture disguised as a participatory patient-led initiative. Lawyer and commentator on genetic testing, Daniel Vorhaus (2012) observed that it was a surprising move for the company to apply for this patent, which is of secondary importance to its most valuable asset: 'an engaged, enthusiastic and growing community of customers-qua-research participants who, provided 23andMe can keep from alienating too many of them, represent something much more unique, and inventive, than US Patent number 8,187,811'. The controversy that the patent application evoked highlights the fragility of trust relations in this context. As Sigrid Sterckx *et al.* (2013: 5) have suggested 'what undermined trust was not so much the profit motive but rather the fact that the company did not provide any clear indication to consumers that it was seeking patents on its discoveries'. As internet users become increasingly aware of the business practices behind sites (for example, in the highly-publicised dispute about properly informing customers about privacy policies and settings on the social networking site Facebook), maintaining trust amid growing consumer scepticism (e.g. through information strategies that demonstrate transparency in practice) will remain important.

Conclusion

There is a growing interest in consumer involvement in medical research (Tutton and Prainsack, 2011), with self-reported data being used by an increasing number of online health groups such as PatientsLikeMe (Allison, 2009; Wicks *et al.*, 2011) and patients using the internet to search for research trials in which to become involved. Medical research relies increasingly on networks of data and collections of tissues stored by research institutions (Lipworth *et al.*, 2011). As the internet is further incorporated into medical research designs, further iterations of online participation in medical research will emerge. 23andMe provides a rich example of what is celebrated as web-based, revolutionary research, utilising a variety of online tools to facilitate participation in genetic research.

In this chapter, we have argued that 23andMe uses various internet platforms to construct an 'empowering' participatory culture, drawing on the democratising potential of the internet and personal genomics. 23andMe attempts to slip effortlessly between commercial and gift exchange, between selling a service and encouraging, even celebrating, research participation. The consumer-participant is presented as offering a saliva sample and personal information in exchange for gifts. Gift exchange implies social bonds which are integral to 23andMe's research method which relies on aggregated genotypic and phenotypic data from a loyal re-contactable cohort. More altruistic notions of participation and gift exchange are used by the company to draw attention away from what we have suggested is a form of free labour, contributing information on the internet through completing the surveys, and clinical labour, submitting the saliva sample for analysis. This free, clinical labour helped the company to build a valuable research and profit-making resource. While 23andMe did work, in terms of organising the analytical and research network and providing a platform for exchange, it is work that added economic value to the 'gifts' offered by customers, value which benefited the company.

Often celebrated as an innovative means of empowerment and democratisation, in this chapter we have thus offered a more critical stance towards consumers' online participation in such research activities. We have shown that slippages are made easily between commercial exchange and gift exchange, in order for the company to enact a feel-good sense of reciprocity and social ties. We follow in the footsteps of internet studies scholars who are interested in the paradoxical nature of internet participation, and who highlight the important synergies between participatory activities and revenue generation (Goldberg, 2011; Proulx *et al.*, 2011: 22). We recognise that participation practices, technologies and markets are intimately connected, and that online participation has an inherent economic quality (Goldberg, 2011: 744).

It is very likely that 23andMe research will have an impact on how medical research is conducted in the future (Tutton and Prainsack, 2011: 2), and further examples such as the Personal Genome Project and the blog Genomes Unzipped show how the internet is shifting genetic research in new directions. The internet changes the nature of research questions asked, ethical processes, the meaning of participation, consent, trust, and research dissemination. Research participants potentially have access to their raw data online and can personalise the results of the genetic research in which they have been involved, something currently debated and under-realised in more traditional medical research (Lipworth *et al.*, 2011: 799). Trust in the self-reported data of individuals about their own health behaviour, rather than their medical records, as well as sharing results so quickly with participants, also changes the nature of medical research, possibly fostering new kinds of relations of trust between research participants and researchers. Self-reported data acknowledge lay knowledge about one's body and healthcare experiences, yet are often criticised by scientific and medical researchers who believe they are unreliable (Arnquist, 2009; Prainsack, 2011). By showing trust in self-reported data, in the individual as a source of information about their own health behaviour and status, rather than the medical record produced by clinicians, these practices foster new ways of thinking about the relations between research participants and researchers. The internet is also fostering new ways of consenting individuals to participate in research, including such approaches as 'dynamic consent' using digital communication to keep research participants informed and engaged with research (an approach that shares some features with the 23andMe notion of a longitudinally engaged research cohort; e.g. Kaye *et al.*, 2014; Wee, 2013). Dynamic consent, as opposed to the traditional paper-based, one-off consent procedure for participation in research, involves recontacting research participants each time new research is proposed to use their data, allowing participants to keep abreast of the science and to make decisions about future participation in research using their data or samples. It makes use of digital media for this ongoing communication.

In this chapter, we have brought together two bodies of literature regarding internet participation and medical research participation, and an analysis of 23andMe web material, to contribute towards a critique of this emerging area of online participation in genetic research. We have focused on the *representation* of these cultural practices, using a commercial website as a starting point and our analysis reflects this. It appears that this kind of participation is pleasurable, desirable and possibly even addictive (Brabham, 2010), but we still need to examine why people participate, and how these motivations compare to other online and medical research participatory practices. We also need to learn more about how consumers understand the information they are sharing, and the consequences of their participation, as well as the social, political, geographical, technological and skill-based constraints on these practices (Henwood *et al.*, 2003; Adams, 2010). Questions arise concerning the kinds of subjectivities and collectivities being formed in these contexts that intermingle genetic and non-genetic identities, affecting how users engage with social groups and form social ties. While more research is needed on user practices, we also need to be cautious about how, as social scientists, we use data provided by participants online, particularly if we want to develop a critical analysis of the ways in which genetic testing companies are making use of material provided by participants (see Appendix A).

Ethical questions also arise about the contribution of bodily material that is stored and accessible, raising concerns about identifiability and possible discrimination on the basis of genetics. These are concerns which add to those of sharing increasing amounts of personal information via the internet. How are third parties such as other researchers, pharmaceutical companies, law enforcement and insurance companies to be involved in this kind of research? What will be the fate of 23andMe's patent applications and how will they be enforced? We have already seen that patent applications caused a lot of distrust among users. What are the ethical, political and economic implications of these developments? Finally, what impact will studies such as those performed by 23andMe, using 'messy', or incomplete, self-reported data, have on the gold standard of medical research; the randomised control trial? In summary, we can conclude that personal genomics research will continue to raise important questions about the forms and consequences of engaging people in research, particularly through the internet, highlighting aspects of informational capitalism that are embedded in internet and medical research practices more broadly.

The move toward reliance on self-reported data that this participatory turn requires brings longer-standing issues of trust to the fore. Self-assessment of symptoms, health and illness, and the validity of self-reported data, are not taken on their own in the medical context; they are contextualised in various ways by the medical professional, using instruments, practices, and the application of expert knowledge. This is an inherent tension and one that is at the heart of diagnostic practices, understood as social (Jutel, 2010). Further, medical interviews are structured by power relationships (e.g. Waitzkin, 1991) and some self-reports in the medical context are given more credibility than others. The use of self-reported data in medical surveillance and in medical research has been called into question (Gordon *et al.*, 1993; Smith *et al.*, 2008), particularly in the online, personal genomics context (Hall and Gartner, 2009). This means that trust becomes actively constructed through materials and discourses in the interactions between various actors.

Filled with 'aspirations, promises, expectations, hopes, desires and imaginings' (Brown, 2003: 4), this participatory movement in medical research has been interpreted by many commentators as a move towards more empowered patients (Arnquist, 2009), and part of more democratic healthcare practices already thought to be enabled by the internet more broadly (Piras and Zanutto, 2010: 586). The general argument behind these promises and expectations is that while people were primarily recipients of online health information in the early days of the internet, with the rise of 'web 2.0', people also produce it, by sharing personal healthcare experiences (e.g. in the form of blogs and fora comments) as well as by contributing to various research enterprises, in practices described as crowd-sourcing or open-source research (Arnquist, 2009). In many cases, participating as an individual is linked to benefits for the community, whereby the idea of contributing data and information becomes intertwined with ideals of good citizenship (Adams, 2010) and improved science. Active health citizenship therefore not only entails responsible self-monitoring, self-care (Piras and Zanutto, 2010: 586) and self-tracking, but also self-reporting.

Participation has long been seen as one of the hallmarks of digital culture (Deleuze and Guattari, 1987), but we should be reminded not to confuse the potential for participation with what is currently happening. We need to distinguish between participation as an action that millions of people now engage in every minute of every day from the consequences of those very diverse forms of participation for science, politics and culture. In addition to the empirical and theoretical questions listed above, we need to ask the normative question of whether 'participation' is always good or to be desired. We also need to remember that hopes about the participatory promises of technologies have accompanied all new media, at least since the printing press.

References

23andMe (2008) 'The power of We', available at http://spittoon.23andme.com/2008/01/21/the-power-of-we (accessed 4 November 2011).

23andMe (2009) '23andWE: the first annual update', available at http://spittoon.23andme.com/2009/01/05/23andwe-the-first-annual-update (accessed 22 July 2011).

23andMe (2010) '23andMe Parkinsons research initiative progress update', available at http://spittoon.23andme.com/2010/01/26/23andme-parkinsons-research-initiative-progress-update (accessed 22 July 2011).

23andMe (2011a) 'Guidelines', available at www.23andme.com/you/community/guidelines (accessed 7 July 2011).

23andMe (2011b) 'Privacy', available at www.23andme.com/legal/privacy (accessed 7 July 2011).

23andMe (2011c) 'Consent', available at www.23andme.com/about/consent (accessed 7 July 2011).

23andMe (2011d) '23andMe research findings from you back to you', available at http://spittoon.23andme.com/2011/06/16/23andme-research-findings-from-you-back-to-you (accessed 22 July 2011).

23andMe (2011e) 'Roots into the future', available at http://spittoon.23andme.com/2011/07/26/roots-into-the-future (accessed 4 November 2011).

23andMe (2011f) 'A recipe for disease research give people tools add passion and shake', available at http://spittoon.23andme.com/2011/07/06/a-recipe-for-disease-research-give-people-tools-add-passion-and-shake (accessed 22 July 2011).

23andMe (2015) '23andWe informed consent', available at www.23andme.com/en-eu/about/consent/?version=2.4 (accessed 15 August 2015).

Abadie, R. (2010) *The professional guinea pig: Big pharma and the risky world of human subjects*, Durham, NC: Duke University Press.

Adams, S. (2010) 'Sourcing the crowd for health experiences: Letting the people speak or obliging voice through choice?', in R. Harris, N. Wathen and S. Wyatt (eds),

Configuring health consumers: Health work and the imperative of personal responsibility, Basingstoke: Palgrave Macmillan, pp. 178–193.

Akrich, M. (2010) 'From communities of practice to epistemic communities: Health mobilizations on the internet', *Sociological Research Online*, vol. 15, no. 2, p. 10, available at www.socresonline.org.uk/15/2/10.html.

Allison, M. (2009) 'Can web 2.0 reboot clinical trials?', *Nature Biotechnology*, vol. 27, no. 10, pp. 895–902.

Arnquist, S. (2009) 'Research trove: Patients' online data', *New York Times*, 24 August, p. D1.

Barbrook, R. (2005) 'The hi-tech gift economy', *First Monday*, special issue no. 3, available at http://firstmonday.org/htbin/cgiwrap/bin/ojs/index.php/fm/article/view/1517 (accessed 2 September 2015).

Bergquist, M. and Ljungberg, J. (2001) 'The power of gifts: Organizing social relationships in open source communities', *Information Systems Journal*, vol. 11, no. 4, pp. 305–320.

Brabham, D. C. (2010) 'Moving the crowd at threadless: Motivations for participation in a crowdsourcing application', *Information, Communication and Society*, vol. 13, no. 8, pp. 1122–1145.

Brown, N. (2003) 'Hope against hype: Accountability in biopasts, presents and futures' *Science Studies*, vol. 16, no. 2, pp. 3–21.

Bruns, A. (2008) *Blogs, Wikipedia, Second Life, and beyond: From production to produsage*, New York: Peter Lang.

Callon, M. and Rabeharisoa, V. (2003) 'Research "in the wild" and the shaping of new social identities', *Technology in Society*, vol. 25, no. 2, pp. 193–204.

Callon, M. and Rabeharisoa, V. (2008) 'The growing engagement of emergent concerned groups in political and economic life', *Science, Technology and Human Values*, vol. 33, no. 2, pp. 230–261.

Collins, H. M. and Evans, R. (2002) 'The third wave of science studies', *Social Studies of Science*, vol. 32, no. 2, pp. 235–296.

Deleuze, G. and Guattari, F. (1987) *A thousand plateaus*, trans. B. Massumi, Minneapolis, MN: University of Minnesota Press (originally published in 1980, *Mille plateaux*, Paris: Minuit).

Do, C. B., Tung, J. Y., Dorfman, E., Kiefer, A. K., Drabant, E. M., Francke, U., Mountain, J. L., Goldman, S. M., Tanner, C. M., Langston, J. W., Wojcicki, A. and Eriksson, N. (2011) 'Web-based genome-wide association study identifies two novel loci and a substantial genetic component for Parkinson's Disease', *PLoS Genetics*, vol. 7, no. 6, article e1002141.

Dolgin, E. (2010) 'Personalized investigation', *Nature Medicine*, vol. 16, no. 9, pp. 953–955.

Epstein, S. (2008) 'Patient groups and health movements', in E. J. Hackett, O. Amsterdamska, M. Lynch and J. Wajcman (eds), *The handbook of science and technology studies*, Cambridge, MA: MIT Press, pp. 499–539.

Eriksson, N., Macpherson, J. M., Michael, J., Tung, J. Y., Hon, L. S., Naughton, B., Saxonov, S., Avey, L., Wojcicki, A., Pe'er, I. and Mountain, J. (2010) 'Web-based, participant-driven studies yield novel genetic associations for common traits', *PLoS Genetics*, vol. 6, no. 6, pp. 1–20.

Eysenbach, G. (2008) 'Medicine 2.0: Social networking, collaboration, participation, apomediation, and openness', *Journal of Medical Internet Research*, vol. 10, no. 3, article e22.

Fish, A., Murillo, L. F. R., Nguyen, L., Panofsky, A. and Kelty, C. M. (2011) 'Birds of the internet', *Journal of Cultural Economy*, vol. 4, no. 2, pp. 157–187.

Goetz, T. (2010) 'Sergey Brin's search for a Parkinson's cure' *Wired Magazine*, available at www.wired.com/magazine/2010/06/ff_sergeys_search/all/1 (accessed 2 September 2015).

Goldberg, G. (2011) 'Rethinking the public/virtual sphere: The problem with participation', *New Media and Society*, vol. 13, no. 5, pp. 739–754.

Gordon, N., Hiatt, R. and Lampert, D. (1993) 'Concordance of self-reported data and medical record audit for six cancer screening procedures', *Journal of the National Cancer Institute* vol. 85, no. 7, pp. 566–570.

Granovetter, M. S. (1973) 'The strength of weak ties', *American Journal of Sociology*, vol. 78, no.6, pp. 1360–1380.

Hall, W. and Gartner, C. (2009) 'Direct-to-consumer genome-wide scans: Astrologicogenomics or simple scams?', *The American Journal of Bioethics*, vol. 9, no. 6, pp. 54–56.

Hallowell, N., Cooke, S., Crawford, G., Lucassen, A., Parker, M. and Snowdon, C. (2010) 'An investigation of patients' motivations for their participation in genetics-related research', *Journal of Medical Ethics*, vol. 36, no. 1, pp. 37–45.

Henwood, F., Wyatt, S., Hart, A. and Smith, J. (2003) '"Ignorance is bliss sometimes": Constraints on the emergence of the "informed patient" in the changing landscapes of health information', *Sociology of Health and Illness*, vol. 25, no. 6, pp. 589–607.

Jenkins, H. (2006) *Convergence culture: Where old and new media collide*, New York, NY: New York University Press.

Jordan, T. (2015) *Information politics: Liberation and exploitation in the digital society*, London: Pluto Press.

Jutel, A. (2010) 'Sociology of diagnosis: A preliminary review', *Sociology of Health and Illness*, vol. 31, no. 2, pp. 278–299.

Karaganis, J. (ed.) (2007) *Structures of participation in digital culture*, New York, NY: Social Science Research Council.

Kaye, J., *et al.* (2014) 'Dynamic consent: A patient interface for twenty-first century research networks', *European Journal of Human Genetics*, vol. 23, pp. 141–146.

Kent, J. (2008) 'The fetal tissue economy: From the abortion clinic to the stem cell laboratory', *Social Science and Medicine*, vol. 67, no. 11, pp. 1747–1756.

Langstrup, H. (2011) 'Interpellating patients as users: Patient associations and the project-ness of stem cell research', *Science, Technology and Human Values*, vol. 36, no. 4, pp. 573–594.

Lawrence, A. (2006) '"No personal motive?" Volunteers, biodiversity, and the false dichotomies of participation', *Ethics, Place and Environment*, vol. 9, no. 3, pp. 279–298.

Levina, M. (2010) 'Googling your genes: Personal genomics and the discourse of citizen bioscience in the network age', *Journal of Science Communication*, vol. 9, no. 1, pp. 1–9.

Li, X. (2011) 'Factors influencing the willingness to contribute information to online communities', *New Media and Society*, vol. 13, no. 2, pp. 279–296.

Lipworth, W., Forsyth, R. and Kerridge, I. (2011) 'Tissue donation to biobanks: A review of sociological studies', *Sociology of Health and Illness*, vol. 33, no. 5, pp. 792–811.

McCray, W. P. (2006) 'Amateur scientists, the International Geophysical year, and the ambitions of Fred Whipple', *Isis*, vol. 97, pp. 634–658.

Mauss, M. (1970) *The gift: Forms and functions of exchange in archaic societies*, London: Cohen and West.

Mitchell, R. and Waldby, C. (2010) 'National biobanks: Clinical labor, risk production, and the creation of biovalue', *Science, Technology and Human Values*, vol. 35, no. 3, pp. 330–355.

Molm, L. D. (2010) 'The structure of reciprocity', *Social Psychology Quarterly*, vol. 73, no. 2, pp. 119–131.

Offer, A. (1997) 'Between the gift and the market: The economy of regard', *The Economic History Review*, vol. 50, no. 3, pp. 450–476.

Pálsson, G. (2009a) 'Biosocial relations of production', *Comparative Studies in Society and History*, vol. 51, no.2, pp. 288–313.

Pálsson, G. (2009b) 'Spitting image', *Anthropology Now*, vol.1, no.3, pp. 12–22.

Panofsky, A. (2011) 'Generating sociability to drive science: Patient advocacy organizations and genetics research', *Social Studies of Science*, vol. 41, no. 1, pp. 31–57.

Pearson, E. (2007) 'Digital gifts: Participation and gift exchange in LiveJournal communities', *First Monday*, vol. 12, no. 5, available at http://firstmonday.org/htbin/cgiwrap/bin/ojs/index.php/fm/article/view/1835/1719 (accessed 2 September 2015).

Piras, E. M. and Zanutto, A. (2010) 'Prescriptions, X-rays and grocery lists: Designing a personal health record to support (the invisible work of) health information management in the household', *Computer Supported Cooperative Work*, vol. 19, pp. 585–613.

Prainsack, B. (2011) 'Voting with their mice: Personal genome testing and the 'participatory turn' in disease research', *Accountability in Research*, vol. 18, no. 3, pp. 132–147.

Prainsack, B. and Wolinsky, H. (2010) 'Direct-to-consumer genome testing: Opportunities for pharmacogenetic research?' *Pharmacogenomics*, vol. 11, no. 5, pp. 651–655.

Proulx, S., Heaton, L. Jane Kwok Choon, M. and Millette, M. (2011) 'Paradoxical empowerment of *produsers* in the context of informational capitalism', *New Review of Hypermedia and Multimedia*, vol. 17, no. 1, pp. 9–29.

Rabeharisoa, V., Moriera, T., and Akrich, M. (2014) 'Evidence-based activism: Patients', users' and activists' groups in knowledge society introduction', *Biosocieties*, vol. 9, pp. 111–128.

Rheingold, H. (2002) *Smart mobs: The next social revolution*, New York, NY: Basic Books.

Saxena, V. (2015) '23andMe's $60M deal with Genentech shows an alternative path forward for diagnostics companies', available at www.fiercemedicaldevices.com/story/23andmes-60m-deal-genentech-shows-alternative-path-forward-diagnostics-comp/2015-01-08 (accessed 20 August 2015).

Schäfer, M. T. (2011) *Bastard culture! How user participation transforms cultural production*, Amsterdam: Amsterdam University Press.

Shapin, S. and Schaffer, S. (1985) *Leviathan and the air-pump: Hobbes, Boyle, and the experimental life*, Princeton, NJ: Princeton University Press.

Shaw, R. (2012) 'Thanking and reciprocating under the New Zealand organ donation system', *Health*, vol. 16, no. 3, pp. 298–313.

Smith, B., Chu, L. K., Smith, T. C., Amoroso, P. J., Boyko, E. J., Hooper, T. I, Gackstetter, G. D., Ryan, M. A. and the Millennium Cohort Study Team (2008) 'Challenges of self-reported medical conditions and electronic medical records among members of a large military cohort', *BMC Medical Research Methodology*, vol. 8, article 37.

Star, S. L. and Griesemer, J. R. (1989) 'Institutional ecology, "translations" and boundary objects: Amateurs and professionals in Berkeley's Museum of Vertebrate Zoology, 1907–1939', *Social Studies of Science*, vol. 19, no. 3, pp. 387–420.

Sterckx, S., Cockbain, J., Howard, H., Huys, I. and Borry, P. (2013) '"Trust is not something you can reclaim easily": Patenting in the field of direct-to-consumer genetic testing', *Genetics in Medicine*, vol. 15, no. 5, pp. 382–387.

Surowiecki, J. (2004) *The wisdom of crowds: Why the many are smarter than the few and how collective wisdom shapes business, economies, societies and nations*, London: Little Brown.

Terranova, T. (2000) 'Free labor: Producing culture for the digital economy', *Social Text*, vol. 18, no. 2, pp. 33–58.

Terry, S. F. and Terry, P. F. (2011) 'Power to the people: Participant ownership of clinical trial data', *Science Translational Medicine*, vol. 3, no. 69, pp. 1–4.

Tober, D. M. (2001) 'Semen as gift, semen as goods: Reproductive workers and the market in altruism', *Body and Society*, vol. 7, nos. 2-3, pp. 137–160.

Tung, J. Y., Do, C. B., Hinds, D. A., Kiefer, A., Macpherson, J. M., Chowdry, A. B., Francke, U., Naughton, B., Mountain, J., Wojcicki, A. and Eriksson, N. (2011) 'Efficient replication of over 180 genetic associations with self-reported medical data', *Nature Precedings*, available at http://precedings.nature.com/documents/6014/version/2 (accessed 2 September 2015).

Turner, V. (1969) *The ritual process: Structure and anti-structure*, Chicago, IL: Aldine.

Tutton, R. (2002) 'Gift relationships in genetics research', *Science as Culture*, vol. 11, no. 4, pp. 523–542.

Tutton, R. and Prainsack, B. (2011) 'Enterprising or altruistic selves? Making up research subjects in genetics research', *Sociology of Health and Illness*, vol. 33, no. 7, pp. 1081–1095.

Vorhaus, D. (2012) 'Patenting and personal genomics: 23andMe receives its first patent, and plenty of questions', *Genomics Law Report*, 1 June, available at www.genomicslawreport.com/index.php/2012/06/01/patenting-and-personal-genomics-23andme-receives-its-first-patent-and-plenty-of-questions (accessed 31 August 2015).

Waitzkin, H. (1991) *The politics of medical encounters: How patients and doctors deal with social problems*, New Haven, CT: Yale University Press.

Waldby, C. (2002) 'Stem cells, tissue cultures and the production of biovalue', *Health*, vol. 6, no. 3, pp. 305–323.

Wee, R. (2013) 'Dynamic consent in the digital age of biology', *Journal of Primary Health Care*, vol. 5, no. 3, pp. 259–261.

Wicks, P., Vaughan, T. E., Massagli, M. P. and Heywood, J. (2011) 'Accelerated clinical discovery using self-reported patient data collected online and a patient-matching algorithm', *Nature Biotechnology*, vol. 29, no. 5, pp. 411–414.

Williams, B., Entwistle, V. Haddow, G. and Wells, M. (2008) 'Promoting research participation: Why not advertise altruism?', *Social Science and Medicine*, vol. 66, no.7, pp. 1451–1456.

5 Controversy

In this chapter, we examine online spaces concerning schizophrenia genetics, a highly contested area of science in which genetics has long played an inconclusive role. We analyse web material from DTC genetic testing companies, focusing on the representation of scientific resources. Selling genetic tests online is itself controversial, and we discuss that below, but our main focus is on how DTC genetic testing companies make use of and represent scientific claims about schizophrenia genetics. The use of controversial scientific claims by these companies has gone some way towards both raising their profile, and positioning DTC genetic testing products as unreliable. Rather than taking sides in these debates, in this chapter we critically examine how different internet platforms affect how scientific controversies unfold. The internet is a fruitful site of investigation of scientific controversy, as it is a technology that is simultaneously content, medium and research infrastructure.

We find that scientific resources are being cited and represented across different platforms of DTC genetic testing companies. They are cited strategically to present a stabilised version of schizophrenia genetics on the main websites of the companies. On the blogs of the same companies, however, science is deployed in a more nuanced way to present a more uncertain (although always hopeful) representation of science. The representations overlap with our findings concerning uses of determinism, discussed in Chapter 1. One would not *a priori* expect to find controversy on commercial websites aiming to sell products. Yet we found traces of the controversies about schizophrenia genetics across these platforms. The controversial nature of the science lends itself to multiple ways of citing and representing resources, and the availability of diverse online spaces enables the practices behind this work to become visible in new ways, both to researchers and to social actors. We argue that, not only do these online spaces make scientific controversy more visible to a wider range of people, they also play a role in the production of knowledge, a role that we argue should be opened up further for critical examination.

In this chapter, we first review the complex and controversial area of schizophrenia genetics, and then outline why controversies are of such interest to social scientists interested in the social and political aspects of science more generally. The central part of the chapter focuses on our analysis of the material we found on the commercial websites and their related blogs, and the differences between these different platforms. In the final section, we draw attention to how the DTC genetic testing companies deploy highly genetically deterministic discourses and at the same time acknowledge the uncertainty surrounding schizophrenia genetics.

Schizophrenia genetics

Schizophrenia is a mental illness characterised by severe psychosis, with clinical symptoms of hallucinations, delusions and interference with thought processes. The disorder is chronic and can be marked by apathy and social isolation. Schizophrenia has a prevalence of 1 per cent in the general population. Since the early twentieth century, when schizophrenia was first labelled, a familial aspect has been suspected. While schizophrenia is known to be highly heritable, with an estimate between 80 and 90 per cent, scientists have struggled to reach consensus about the genetic basis for the condition (Lewontin, 1991; Hedgecoe, 2001).

As technologies of genetic analysis have evolved, the methods of searching for genetic associations with schizophrenia have changed from the early focus on twin and adoption studies. More prevalent in the early twenty-first century are reports of genome-wide association studies (GWAS) which can detect genes with small effects by scanning the whole genome in large study populations; the results of research studying gene and environment interactions; and rare and *de novo* mutations (Burmeister *et al.*, 2008; Maiti *et al.*, 2011; Tienari *et al.*, 2004; Walsh *et al.*, 2008). In a move from 'meta-analysis' to 'mega-analysis', research is being conducted by well-funded large consortia that amalgamate databases across multiple research institutions in the hope of finding rare genetic associations for schizophrenia. A study from the Schizophrenia Psychiatric Genome-Wide Association Study Consortium (2011) combined GWAS data from 17 separate studies conducted in 11 countries, involving almost 10,000 cases and over 12,000 controls. A study published in *Molecular Psychiatry* in 2012 brought together data from these GWAS, as well as results concerning linkages, copy number variants, gene expression (from human post-mortem samples, cell lines, or blood samples), and animal model studies of schizophrenia (GenomeWeb, 2012).

Controversies have plagued this continually evolving field, including its association with eugenics, the role of twin and adoption studies in understanding the genetic basis of mental illnesses (Hedgecoe, 2001) and the failure of genetic linkage studies to find 'genes for' schizophrenia (Arribas-Allyon and Bartlett, 2010). Despite the series of 'landmark' research papers mentioned above, as of this writing there is no consensus on identifying a precise genetic cause of schizophrenia (Duncan and Keller, 2011). Concern is raised in academic journals, in newspapers, and in blogs, about the lack of replication of research findings and whether each new study ever reveals anything really novel. Some believe that the difficulties lie in an unclear definition of the schizophrenia phenotype (Frazzetto, 2009) that is based on clinical examination and diagnostic criteria in the *Diagnostic and Statistical Manual of Mental Disorders* or the *International*

Classification of Disorders (Burmeister *et al.*, 2008: 529). These diagnostic criteria are themselves controversial, in the clinic as well as in research (Hedgecoe, 2001). Considering this diagnostic uncertainty, some researchers advocate for research into endophenotypes, or components of the disease, such as anxiety or psychosis, rather than the disease itself, recognising that genetic variants do not map neatly onto current diagnostic categories (Insel and Wang, 2010). Endophenotype research, adopted by one of the DTC genetic testing companies discussed below, is argued however to be just another framework for the same project of attempting to understand the genetic basis of schizophrenia (Arribas-Allyon and Bartlett, 2010).

Schizophrenia genetics remains a controversial area of research (Brzustowicz and Freedman, 2011; Burmeister *et al.*, 2008; Mitchell *et al.*, 2010). Following all of the controversies in this scientific field is beyond the scope of this chapter; however it is important to locate our argument within this contentious area of scientific research related to schizophrenia genetics as well as within the controversial nature of internet-mediated healthcare and scientific practice. In the next section, we review some of the history of 'controversy studies', before moving on to present how we found controversies to play out on the DTC genetic testing company websites.

Controversy goes online

Controversies have long been of interest to social scientists engaged with the social, cultural, moral and political aspects of medicine, science and technology. Controversies are considered interesting because they offer insight into the processes by which facts become stable, before science becomes 'normal' (Latour, 1987); scholars have been interested in, among other things, how research findings such as those in genetics become stabilised as 'facts' about human biology (M'Chareck, 2013). Decades of scholarship have shown empirically that a vast array of actors are involved in scientific controversies, not only between scientific peers (Collins, 1975, 2004; Shapin and Schaffer, 1985; MacKenzie, 1990) but also involving other actors, from patients and their advocates (Epstein, 2008) to sheep farmers (Wynne, 1992) and bee keepers (Suryanarayanan and Kleinman, 2013), for example. The outcome of controversies matter to people in a range of positions relative to the production of science, and this is certainly the case in the production of genetic science, in which the findings purport to tell us important things about human biology and human health. Social scientists find that actors draw on various forms of experience and expertise to position themselves within their particular area of contestation, shaping how the controversies unfold and what becomes established as fact.

Technologies of communication also play a role in how controversies take shape. Historical examples can be found in the information infrastructure of postal systems in the seventeenth and eighteenth centuries, enabling the exchange of public and private correspondence between scientific 'men of letters' (Bowker *et al.*, 2010: 104) or the mass circulation of peer-reviewed journals in the mid-nineteenth century (Lightman, 2011). As the distribution patterns of scientific knowledge exchange widened with the development of these communication technologies, alongside developments in transportation, communication within the scientific community became, as Geoffrey Bowker and colleagues (2010: 104) write, 'no longer two-way, but *n*-way', implying a multiplicity of possible directions, a move that would be strengthened by open access to scientific publications. We can also look to controversies that have more directly involved lay people (see for example Epstein, 2008, on the involvement of patient groups in health movements, as well as the discussion of lay involvement in scientific controversies in Persson and Welin, 2008).

As discussed more extensively in both Chapter 1 and Appendix A, we start from the assumption that new technologies of communication support (or reproduce) existing forms of exchange while also creating new sites for scientific controversy. We take the position that as a site of representation the internet is not neutral but mediates that representation and knowledge production by, at least, providing alternative sites for representation. The 'internet' is far from monolithic, comprising a multitude of pages, links, media, and platforms, each with their own meanings, practices and possibilities.

As discussed above, we focus on a specific scientific topic, schizophrenia genetics, and how it is discussed in particular internet spaces. Schizophrenia genetic research itself is a particularly controversial area of medical science that has already captured the attention of STS scholars (Hedgecoe, 2001; Rabeharisoa and Bourret, 2009; Arribas-Allyon and Bartlett, 2010). As already discussed, new directions in schizophrenia research call for 'polyevidence' studies or mega-analyses (e.g. Schizophrenia Psychiatric Genome-Wide Association Study Consortium, 2011), which draw together singular studies and meta-analyses, pulling into alignment evidence from research conducted using similar or different methodologies, some including cross-species databases, and much of which uses the internet as a medium of communication and work. The commercial marketing of tests on the basis of this research is, if anything, even more contentious (Brzustowicz and Freedman, 2011; Burmeister *et al.*, 2008; Couzin, 2008; Mitchell *et al.*, 2010), an issue we find to be significant in the representation practices of DTC genetic testing companies.

While social scientists have examined various contexts in which scientific knowledge is played out, few have focused specifically on the ways in which scientific knowledge is represented and produced across different internet platforms. There has been a recent focus in STS on the role of the internet in database management and knowledge production (Bowker, 2000; Hine, 2006; Leonelli, 2012). Such work examines data-based exchanges between scientists and others involved in scientific work. We complement this study of the internet in science by looking at exchanges occurring outside the 'core-set' (Collins and Evans, 2002) of schizophrenia genetic science, across public internet platforms accessed and constructed by users with a wide range of expertise. We suggest that a new way of thinking about controversy outside of the 'core set' is in its multiple, often conflicting representations.

Spaces of contestation, controversy and debate in regards to psychiatric illness have largely been restricted to physical locations such as clinical meeting rooms (Spandler, 2009), classification manuals (George, Whitehouse and Ballenger, 2011; Kawa and Giordano, 2012), and specifically in the field of schizophrenia genetics, the clinic, the clinic-laboratory interface (Rabeharisoa and Bourret, 2009) and journal publications (Arribas-Allyon and Bartlett, 2010; Hedgecoe, 2001). Researchers have queried whether the internet will allow room for new forms of 'psychiatric contention' to develop (Spandler, 2009: 678), and we address this by looking at what happens when schizophrenia genetics goes online, picking up the theme of changing temporal and spatial relations addressed in Chapter 1.

We focus on how the technical architecture of the internet shapes the utilisation and representation of knowledge resources, rather than on the content of the research studies. In this way our work differs from that of other researchers who, in the context of psychiatric genetics, have examined how scientific resources are taken up in the clinic (Rabeharisoa and Bourret, 2009), or cited in review articles (Hedgecoe, 2006). We focus on the web presence of companies offering DTC genetic testing, and how research into the genetic basis for schizophrenia is presented and contested by companies selling genetic tests directly to the public. As described more extensively in Appendix A, our methodological approach to the internet aligns with those who consider the infrastructural details of internet technology as important and worthy of analysis (Beaulieu and Simakova, 2006; Bowker *et al.*, 2010; Hine, 2006; Wouters *et al.*, 2013). For this reason we collected web material from a range of platforms, looking at infrastructural details such as hyperlinks, which provide insight into how websites act as spaces for sharing and circulating scientific resources (Beaulieu, 2005), as well as examining where decisions concerning the controversy are made more visible. The very idea of selling genetic tests via the internet provoked strong reactions, and the next section addresses some of those.

Selling genetic tests online for schizophrenia

The origins of the DTC genetic testing industry were discussed in Chapter 1. To recap, in 2011, more than 50 companies were registered to sell such tests, mostly in the US but also Iceland, and were beginning to appear in Australia, Canada, UK, Singapore and Ireland (Dvoskin and Kaufman, 2011; see also Genetics and Public Policy Center, 2010, for a published list of 30 companies which were reported in 2010).

From its start, there was controversy concerning the DTC genetic testing industry among many in the medical and scientific communities. Arguments against selling genetic tests via the internet included the following: the genetic information upon which the tests are based is unreliable; the clinical utility of the tests is limited; the genetic information is most often provided without the involvement of a medical practitioner or genetic counsellor (this was initially the case although the industry has mediated these practices somewhat – we discuss this in Chapter 3); the tests are based on risk variants which are poorly under-stood by the scientific community; and the companies are largely unregulated (Parliamentary Office of Science and Technology, 2012; Lerner-Ellis, Ellis and Green, 2013). Concerns about consistency of test results were raised after vari-ations were uncovered in the results made for individuals purchasing tests from different companies (Trapp, 2010). Many members and organisations within scientific and medical communities have expressed their wariness about DTC genetic testing companies, and what they view as the risks that this information may have for individuals, who may (mis)understand, (mis)interpret and have difficulties coping with their genetic information (American Congress of Obstetricians and Gynecologists, 2008; Couzin, 2008; Hudson *et al.*, 2007; National Society of Genetic Counselors, 2010). However, others have argued that DTC genetic testing is a way to empower consumers, who are now able to take their genetic information into their own hands (Harvey, 2010), outside the strictures of the clinic. We wanted to see how 'empowerment' might play out in the controversial (for both scientific and social reasons) arena of schizophrenia genetics.

Some commentators in medical and science journals (Braff and Freedman, 2008; Burmeister *et al.*, 2008) consider DTC genetic testing for psychiatric illness as a particularly problematic target for the industry, because of the 'prematurity' of the science. A somewhat paternalistic concern comes across in many of these critiques (as well as some boundary maintenance between 'good' and 'bad' science), about consumers being misled and misinformed by the test results. Deploying a less paternalistic tone, Arribas-Allyon, Sarangi and Clarke (2011) argue that DTC genetic testing for genetic susceptibility to psychiatric conditions shifts the burden of responsibility to clinicians and patients for recognising the complexity of the genetics, and the limited predictability of the test. As we show below, on the company website, consumers of these products are given only partial glimpses of the science, which is selected and represented in specific ways in order to sell the tests.

The direct-to-consumer genetic testing companies

The market for psychiatric genetic tests has proved to be volatile, reflecting the uncertainty of the science regarding the diagnosis and treatment of schizophrenia and other illnesses. Pharmaceutical companies that once invested in this area have pulled out after not seeing any advances (Abbott, 2010), and the DTC genetic testing company Neuromark removed their tests for psychiatric conditions from the market, after initially offering them. Of the 20 websites we found in 2011 sell-ing tests for mental illnesses, three offered genetic tests for schizophrenia as part of a broader 'health and illness' package (23andMe, MapMyGene, Lumigenix); and two engaged in research on psychiatric conditions but did not sell tests directly to consumers. The website of each company at the time of analysis is discussed below, focusing on how scientific resources were utilised by each company.

23andMe remains one of the most well-known DTC genetic testing companies. Registered in the US in 2007, at the time of our main analysis in 2011, the internet-based company offered consumers an array of genetic tests for 234 disease risks, traits and pharmacological responses, as well as for ancestry. The page dedicated to schizophrenia offered a brief description of symptoms, risk factors and statistics, with mention that the disease is 'thought to be highly heritable'. There was no mention that only a small part of the heritability of schizophrenia has been studied genetically, and that most remains unexamined in terms of the influence of non-genetic effects.

The 23andMe sample report for schizophrenia implied that two markers of the disease were tested for, based on preliminary research, which was described (via a hyperlink) as results from studies that had yet to be confirmed by the scientific community and were possibly contradictory. The sample report provided details and further hyperlinks to PubMed abstracts of the two studies upon which the genetic marker evidence was based. The first article, from the *Journal of Human Genetics*, was a Japanese study of 2000 people diagnosed with schizophrenia and 2000 with no personal/family history of mental illness, and reported no replication studies or contrary studies. The second cited study, from *Human Molecular Genetics*, reported that 800 men with schizophrenia were compared with 2000 healthy men, which again had no replications or contrary studies, this time with applicable ethnicities stated as 'European'. 23andMe acknowledged that this second study examined women but did not find an association.

MapMyGene, a Singapore-based company, at the time of analysis, offered genetic testing for disease susceptibility as well as for 'inborn talent'. The website was aimed at a bilingual audience, with brochures about its genetic testing services provided in English and Chinese. MapMyGene included schizophrenia in its list of 120 diseases detectable by its DNA sequencing disease susceptibility gene test, although information regarding the specific markers was not provided.

While no resources from scientific journals were provided, on a webpage dedicated to 'Quotes from professionals in the field', expert commentaries about genetic testing for schizophrenia evoked genetic determinist arguments and advocated early intervention. For example, the website referred to a 2007 commentary written by James Watson, one of the identifiers of the structure of DNA, in the British newspaper *The Independent*, which suggested that Watson's drive for bringing 'the human genome into existence', was his son's suffering from schizophrenia, the origin of which Watson came to believe 'lay in his genes'.

Lumigenix was launched in Australia in January 2011 as a company jointly funded by seed money from the federal Australian Government and private equity. It partnered with the Mayo Clinic, Illumina and the Australian Genome Research Facility. At the time of analysis, two levels of genetic testing were offered by the company: an introductory test which examined an individual's risk for 76 diseases, and a more comprehensive test examining 81 diseases and providing updates as new research findings become available. Prices of the Lumigenix tests were displayed in US dollars, and media links provided to

Australian television shows, suggesting the company was targeting both American and Australian markets.

Lumigenix tested for schizophrenia from five, unspecified, single nucleotide polymorphisms (SNPs). A sample report was provided with information about symptoms, causes, risk factors, complications, treatment, diagnosis and prevention of schizophrenia. Lumigenix did not provide links to any scientific publications on the schizophrenia webpages, but did provide links to Mayo Clinic resources. Lumigenix claimed that its links to the 'world-renowned Mayo Clinic' allowed it to 'deliver the most accurate and appropriate peer-reviewed medical content', based on 'the experience and knowledge of more than 3,400 physicians and scientists of Mayo Clinic'.

SureGene, an American company, did not sell genetic tests for schizophrenia, but was developing a test for schizophrenia based upon its own scientific research (Couzin, 2008). There were no hyperlinks to its existing published research on the website. On the page representing its research, SureGene claimed that 'we are redefining mental illness by focusing on endophenotypes'. SureGene conducted research on endophenotypes such as obsessiveness, mania and paranoia. Further online searching revealed that this company had applied for various patents in relation to genetic markers for schizophrenia and antipsychotic response.

DeCODE, an Icelandic research group with a commercial genetic testing component called DeCODEMe, claimed to have had success in its genetic research about schizophrenia, having being involved in this area for some time. Numerous research articles have been published in high-profile journals such as *Nature*. DeCODEMe applied for a patent in May 2011 related to genetic markers for schizophrenia, but at the time of analysis did not sell a test for the disease.

Strategic use of scientific resources on the websites

The first three DTC genetic testing companies listed above referenced a variety of scientific resources including research studies published in peer-reviewed journals (23andMe), 'legitimate' institutions (e.g. Mayo Clinic information by Lumigenix) and quoted commentary in other media (MapMyGene). SureGene and DeCODE, which did not offer tests for schizophrenia, chose not to draw on their own published research. For those offering testing for schizophrenia, we suggest that resources were used strategically in two main ways, namely to reinforce genetic determinism and to simplify what is a very complex scientific debate.

First, resources were used to reinforce genetic deterministic viewpoints (see also Chapter 1). Commentaries on MapMyGene, and the PubMed articles emphasised a genetically deterministic view of how genes affect mental health (implying genetic causation), a narrative, we argue, the companies rely upon in order to market their product. While Lumigenix acknowledged the influence of environmental factors in the development of schizophrenia, the surrounding text nonetheless reinforced the genetic underpinnings of the disease and the potential to avert illness through early intervention, itself implying a known or knowable causal route.

Second, by simplifying genetic associations, the companies represented a less complex picture of schizophrenia aetiology than other online sources such as Wikipedia (see Wyatt, Harris and Kelly, 2016) or close reading of scientific papers. Although adding more genes does not mean more accurate information, since complex gene interactions increase the difficulty of interpretation (Arribas-Allyon, Sarangi and Clarke, 2011), the companies were nonetheless deliberately reducing complexity through their selective and strategic use of genetic markers and scientific resources. Selling a test based on only two or five genetic markers, when many more have been identified within the scientific literature, reduces complexity. Both the genetic determinism narrative (see Chapter 1) and the reduction of complexity serve to reinforce certainty and provide the impression of stable facts. Although 23andMe acknowledges, through a hyperlink, the preliminary nature of the research reports upon which the schizophrenia genetic marker information was based, this doubt was otherwise masked by the glossy and well-designed sample report, which referred to only two scientific articles, a simplistic and certain representation of the science.

These findings confirm what others have found regarding psychiatric genetic testing, concerning genetic determinism, certainty and complexity. The genetic testing possibilities for mental illnesses such as schizophrenia are widely believed to be overstated (Owen, McGuffin and Gottesman, 2003). Arribas-Allyon and colleagues (2011: 519) note that 'when commercial actors seek to profit from the results of molecular research the public are sold simple genetics, not the complexity so meticulously constructed in review papers' and point out that the scientific community utilises the complexity of research in order to stress the lack of clinical utility of the simplified genetic tests. In their analysis of psychiatric genetics, Braff and Freedman (2008) consider that the reduced complexity with limited predictability of tests may be harmful to patients.

These are certainly considerations to keep in mind; however, we found that the stable and static representation of schizophrenia genetics sold to consumers visiting the company websites changed when discussions of the science were taken to different platforms. When discussions moved to company blogs, a more nuanced representation of schizophrenia genetic science appeared, with more complicated understandings of the science presented by the same actors simultaneously. We discuss this below.

Uncertainty in the blogs

Many of the DTC genetic testing companies we examined used a variety of social media platforms in order to engage with consumers, such as blogs, Twitter and YouTube. The various platforms they used appeared to have different, although potentially overlapping, users in mind than those accessing their main page. The internet enabled different versions of the science to be presented to consumers simultaneously. Blogs in particular were used by companies in order to share web material which promoted their products. Blogs are characterised by the publication of various kinds of content (posts) in reverse chronological order, including hyperlinks, images and written text, as well as archives of posts and search functions (Siles, 2011). Blog posts and comments are shaped by the technical infrastructure of the blogging format, and the content added by both administrators and commenters.

Blogging platforms were used by genetic testing companies as a way to communicate with visitors to their sites. Among the websites we examined, 23andMe excelled at maintaining its blog as an integral part of its online presence, using it to represent a complex picture of schizophrenia genetic science, very different from the certainty presented on the main website. For example, a blog post in 2008 discussed how GWAS, the source of most of the data that 23andMe uses, 'may not be the way to go' in schizophrenia research. Discussing an article published by *Science*, the post described how the authors of the paper suggest that genetic predisposition to schizophrenia is caused by structural variations, instead of the SNPs for which the company tests, a suggestion that directly undermined claims made elsewhere on the site about the usefulness of a genetic test. Another Spittoon blog post reported on a study in *Nature Genetics* where:

> Unfortunately, the variant ultimately found to have the strongest association with schizophrenia – rs1344706 – is not included in *23andMe*'s database … These studies suggest that very rare gene mutations might play more of a role in the disease than had previously been supposed. That's valuable information for scientists, and may explain why the genetics of schizophrenia have been so difficult to figure out. But it also suggests that it will take much more research to understand the genetic risk factors underlying schizophrenia than many other diseases.

In these blog discussions, 23andMe presented a science which was much more unstable than the science represented on the website. In doing this, 23andMe was simultaneously presenting genetic deterministic certainty on one platform, and uncertainty cloaked in a promissory, utopian narrative, on another. There may be many reasons for doing this, e.g. to avoid litigation, or to engage in regulatory debates (Curnutte and Testa, 2012), or to highlight overlooked dimensions of the value of being genetically tested (Groves and Tutton, 2013).

Other DTC genetic testing companies similarly used blogs in order to present alternative versions of the science than those presented on their main websites. While DeCODEMe did not sell a test for schizophrenia, it did use its blog to share the promises of its research in this area. In July 2008, a DeCODEMe blog post declared that findings from its research 'may provide the foundation for a test to complement standard clinical diagnosis, potentially enabling earlier intervention and treatment'. The results of its self-proclaimed 'spectacular' study were released in *Nature* in July 2009. As outlined above however, the DeCODEMe website made no claims about schizophrenia genetic testing, and the blog post remained a reminder of the economy of hope (Morrison, 2012) tied into DTC genetic testing, embedded, although not so visibly, on the website. The blog enabled the company to share the research, without bringing into question the certainty being sold on its main website.

In summary, our analysis of DTC genetic testing online spaces shows that rather than purely being a case of stabilisation and selective marketing, the internet enabled the presence of co-existing representations of scientific knowledge. We found that the companies certainly presented a simplistic, genetically deterministic narrative of schizophrenia genetics on their websites, but we also found the presentation of a more uncertain picture of the science on other platforms available to them. Although wrapped in promissory and utopian dressing, the alternative versions we analysed nonetheless demonstrate how the companies can make use of other internet platforms to explore controversy in ways that do not necessarily detract from the simple marketing message on their websites. In the next section, we offer a more detailed examination of what the different company platforms mean for the representation and production of knowledge.

Controversy in action: citation and production of knowledge

Schizophrenia genetic science is represented in multiple ways across different internet platforms. Two different representations of schizophrenia genetics are provided by genetic testing companies, through their varying use and interpretation of resources across multiple platforms. The different platforms used by genetic testing companies also presumably have different (although again overlapping) users in mind. The websites are aimed primarily at consumers buying the test, whereas the blog is directed to those more interested in genetics research and the activities of the company, such as potential research participants (who may simultaneously be consumers). It is also important for the companies to maintain some credibility in regards to the science, needing to be seen to be engaging with current research. Groves and Tutton (2013) describe how genetic testing companies are always walking a tightrope between regulation and innovation, between wanting to maintain some degree of scientific legitimacy and needing to sell tests to consumers. Our analysis showed that a company like 23andMe can both participate in the complexities of controversy, and also attempt to stabilise the controversy in order to deliver a product to their consumers (hence the sale of a test based on two genetic markers, from research conducted five years previously). While the websites presented a stable science, the blogs showed evidence of more complex, although always promissory, understandings of scientific knowledge. It is the very nature of this controversial science which enables a DTC genetic testing company to 'freeze' or stabilise the science in two static genetic markers, as the lack of consensus on genetic association means that these markers, while not representing the full range of genetic association, are nonetheless recognised by some researchers as showing a link with the disease in some populations. The controversial nature of schizophrenia genetics thus allows these multiple versions of the science to co-exist.

The internet is clearly an important medium for the exchange of scientific information among scientists, and also between science, industry, government and the public. Looking at the ways in which controversy appears across different online spaces helps to open the black box of the internet itself, and to challenge deterministic assumptions (see Chapter 1). Our analysis reveals both stabilisation practices and representations of controversy as potentially resolvable promissory uncertainty, a temporary state. The infrastructure of the internet enabled these processes to be made more visible, an infrastructure that facilitates new relationships and practices. We found evidence, particularly in the company blogs, of new kinds of interactions between patients, scientists, medical professionals and others, negotiating expertise and evidence, in ways which have not been previously possible in hospitals, clinics, laboratories, and other places where the classification, diagnosis and treatment of disease have been discussed.

When sociologists of science began studying controversies in the 1970s, they studied them as experiments that opened up the formal hard shell of science to expose the 'soft social inside filled with seeds of everyday thought' (Collins and Evans, 2002: 248). Controversies have always been enabled and enacted through the means of communication technologies, although we argue that the internet facilitates this process, by making those 'everyday thoughts' visible in ways which were not previously possible and by bringing a wider range of actors into the controversy. The internet thus offers a more public viewing of 'controversy in action', of the ways in which actors select and use resources, that differs from the more closed-shop controversy work that goes into discussing the clinical relevance of genetic findings behind the closed doors of expert group meetings (Rabeharisoa and Bourret, 2009).

Different versions of schizophrenia genetics were enacted online through partial presentation of resources. We have seen in the online spaces discussed above, that actors can utilise varied and often creative understandings of 'citation'. While most actors drew upon peer-reviewed journal articles (MapMyGene and Lumigenix show some exceptions), they were used in different ways. This *ad hoc* approach was partly a result of the sheer number of unreplicated studies published in peer-reviewed journals, the ever-changing review articles in this area of science in top journals, and the constant stream of 'breakthroughs'. Many of the genetic research papers that were hyperlinked required subscriptions in order to access them. Structural barriers therefore existed for those who did not have access to these resources. In many ways, however, the resource at the end of the hyperlink is not itself the most important element, but rather it is the presence of the hyperlink that provides credibility. It functions not only to direct the user to the resource, but also as a way of signalling legitimacy by creating alliances which may not necessarily be two-, or even n-way, but often one-way. This becomes important to consider more carefully, when one realises that consumers may only be linking to paper abstracts as evidence, within which the complexities and limitations presented in a scientific paper are not always evident.

Many selective versions of schizophrenia genetics were represented in the online spaces we examined. In many ways, this is not surprising, because the definition, causes, diagnosis and treatment of schizophrenia have long been and continue to be deeply controversial. But in other ways, it is very surprising because companies selling products do not usually make visible the scientific controversies that might render their products unsalable or less desirable. Below the surface of opening home pages, we observed debate and dissent. But we want to go further, and consider these not only as places where knowledge is distributed and knowledge claims are debated but also as places where knowledge is produced. DTC genetic testing companies not only draw on genetic science to undertake testing, but they also engage in research, undertaken through various web 2.0 platforms, and building on the genetic samples people pay to provide. They invite their customers/web page viewers to provide genetic and phenotype data, and thus engage directly in the production of knowledge.

The internet is an important source of information for individuals about health and illness, including schizophrenia. DTC genetic testing companies are not only selling products, they are also engaging in the science, not only in the ways in which they sell their products but also in how they engage with their customers to become sites of knowledge production (Curnutte and Testa, 2012). Three of the companies we examined engaged in research of different kinds: Suregene is a research development company, DeCODE had a strong history of conducting research in schizophrenia genetics and the genetics of other conditions, and 23andMe combines its steadily accumulating database of consumers' genetic data with their self-reported phenotypic data, which it has since used (and sold) for scientific research. In line with the company's 'research 2.0' mantra, 23andMe described and continues to describe these research methodologies as 'participant-led' or 'patient-driven' (Do *et al.*, 2011; Eriksson *et al.*, 2010). Illness experience is actively solicited by 23andMe in order to do research, and thus the self-reported data, about diseases such as schizophrenia, becomes vital data (Wyatt *et al.*, 2013).

In a publication based on its research released on the *Nature Precedings* website, 23andMe reported that it had predicted it would find 0.71 replications for schizophrenia, yet it did not manage to replicate any previously identified genetic associations for schizophrenia after seven attempts. Not only did 23andMe not find any associations for schizophrenia while continuing to sell the test, the company researchers tested for genetic markers which were actually *different* from those upon which they based its commercially available test.

These research activities highlight a further version of schizophrenia genetics that differs from the websites and the blogs. The consequences of how these genetic testing companies engage in research is important to consider because the companies embroiled in psychiatric genetic research have their own commercial, pharmaceutical and patenting ambitions. While companies such as 23andMe proclaim to be at the forefront of new research methods and dissemination practices, they continue to regard publication of their own research in peer-reviewed journals as important. Even though the companies claim to operate outside traditional science, they continue to rely upon its structures and resources for credibility (Curnutte and Testa, 2012).

Conclusion

The multitude of theories, methods, and research studies in the field of schizophrenia genetics means that each representation of the science on the internet platforms we studied is not 'inaccurate', but rather a partial citation or representation of resources, in which material is curated (selected, evaluated and presented). This results not only in the circulation of existing knowledge but also the production of new knowledge. We argue that the internet enables social action around the citation of these resources in ways which were not possible with earlier forms of communication technology, while infrastructural features such as journal subscription fees and editing rights work to constrain engagement with the science. Elsewhere (Wyatt, Harris and Kelly, 2016), we have drawn on the notion of 'curation' to understand how Wikipedia produces knowledge, also about schizophrenia genetics. But Wikipedia works differently from the corporate web presences we have discussed in this chapter, in which people are presumed to be a passive audience of the information provided, or, more importantly people are consumers of the product of DTC genetic testing, or participating in the research activities of the companies (see also Chapter 2).

The internet is well on the way to becoming black boxed, as the inner workings of computers and the means for connecting them are increasingly taken for granted. This only makes it more crucial to pay attention to how the internet affects how patients, carers, scientists and medical professionals understand, interpret and engage with science. As discussed in the Introduction, we suggest that the internet is opening up new c/sites of scientific controversy shaped not only by consumers, patients, scientists, companies and doctors but also by technological infrastructure, allowing new interactions and making actors' engagements with these controversies visible in previously unseen ways. By recognising that different online spaces can and may be used differently by actors, providing different kinds of information about an important topic, our analysis aims to keep the black box open. Numerous social science researchers have broadened the spaces for examining the production of scientific knowledge beyond the laboratory, and in this chapter, we have contributed an analysis of some of the new media spaces in which controversies unfold.

The example of schizophrenia genetics provides insight into the role that the internet plays in contemporary scientific controversies concerning a particular medical condition. Unlike in the clinic, where categories of illness are attempted to be stabilised, or in journal articles, where coherent narratives are constructed, on the internet we see deliberate playing with the instability induced by controversy. The internet allows new spaces (see Chapter 1) for analysis of controversy, each version, representation and argument shaped by actors and the infrastructure of the platforms. While we recognise that the internet allows people, as consumers, potential patients, or those simply curious about science, to engage with science in new ways with new media, we are cautious in celebrating what many regard as the emancipatory, democratic potential of this participatory engagement with genetic science. Instead we have examined how the internet affects and structures the ways in which controversies play out, and how that process sometimes stabilises and sometimes undermines existing knowledge, and sometimes generates new knowledge, all of which may affect how people come to trust (see Chapter 1) both genetic knowledge and the medium by which they acquired that knowledge.

References

Abbott, A. (2010) 'The drug deadlock', *Nature*, vol. 48, pp. 158–159.

American Congress of Obstetricians and Gynecologists (2008) 'ACOG committee opinion no. 409: Direct-to-consumer marketing of genetic testing', *Obstetrics and Gynecology*, vol. 111, no.6, pp. 1493–1494.

Arribas-Allyon, M. and Bartlett, A. (2010) 'Complexity and accountability: the witches' brew of psychiatric genetics', *Social Studies of Science*, vol. 40, no. 4, pp. 499–524.

Arribas-Allyon, M., Sarangi, S. and Clarke, A. (2011) *Genetic testing: Accounts of autonomy, responsibility and blame*, London: Routledge.

Beaulieu, A. (2005) 'Sociable hyperlinks: an ethnographic approach to connectivity', in C. Hine (ed.), *Virtual methods: Issues in social research on the internet*, New York: Berg, pp. 183–197.

Beaulieu, A. and Simakova, E. (2006) 'Textured connectivity: an ethnographic approach to understanding the timescape of hyperlinks', *Cybermetrics: International Journal of Scientometrics, Informetrics and Bibliometrics*, vol. 10, no. 1.

Bowker, G. C. (2000) 'Biodiversity datadiversity', *Social Studies of Science*, vol. 30, no. 5, pp. 643–683.

Bowker, G. C., Baker, K., Millerand, F. and Ribes, D. (2010) 'Towards information infrastructure studies: Ways of knowing in a networked environment', in J. Hunsinger, L. Klastrup and M. Allen (eds), *International handbook of internet research*, Berlin: Springer, pp. 97–118.

Braff, D. and Freedman, R. (2008) 'Clinically responsible genetic testing in neuropsychiatric patients: A bridge too far too soon', *American Journal of Psychiatry* vol. 165, no. 8, pp. 952–955.

Brzustowicz, L. and Freedman, R. (2011) 'Digging more deeply for genetic effects in psychiatric illness', *American Journal of Psychiatry*, vol. 168, no. 10, pp. 1017–1020.

Burmeister, M., *et al.* (2008) 'Psychiatric genetics: Progress amid controversy', *Nature Reviews Genetics*, no. 9 (July), pp. 527–540.

Collins, H. M. (1975) 'The seven sexes: A study in the sociology of a phenomenon, or the replication of experiments in physics', *Sociology*, vol. 9, no. 2, pp. 205–224.

Collins, H. M. (2004) *Gravity's shadow: The search for gravitational waves*, Chicago, IL: University of Chicago Press.

Collins, H. M. and Evans, R. (2002) 'The third wave of science studies', *Social Studies of Science*, vol. 32, no. 2, pp. 235–296.

Couzin, J. (2008) 'Gene tests for psychiatric risk polarize researchers', *Science*, vol. 319, no. 5861, pp. 274–277.

Curnutte, M. and Testa, G. (2012) 'Consuming genomes: Scientific and social innovation in direct-to-consumer genetic testing', *New Genetics and Society*, vol. 31, no. 2, pp. 159–181.

Do, C. B. *et al.* (2011) 'Web-based genome-wide association study identifies two novel loci and a substantial genetic component for Parkinson's Disease', *PLoS Genetics*, vol. 7, no. 6, article e1002141.

Duncan, L. E. and Keller, M. C. (2011) 'A critical review of the first 10 years of candidate gene-by-environment interaction research in psychiatry', *American Journal of Psychiatry*, vol. 168, no. 10, pp. 1041–1049.

Dvoskin, R. and Kaufman, D. (2011) *Direct-to-consumer genetic testing companies*, Baltimore, MD: Genetics and Public Policy Center, Johns Hopkins University, was available at www.dnapolicy.org/pub.reports.php?action=detail&report_id=28 (accessed 17 August 2011; archived at www.webcitation.org/610DDbCns).

Epstein, S. (2008) 'Patient groups and health movements', in E. J. Hackett, O. Amsterdamska, M. Lynch and J. Wajcman (eds), *Handbook of Science and Technology Studies*, Cambridge, MA: MIT Press, pp.499–539.

Eriksson, N., Macpherson, J. M., Tung, J. Y., Hon, L. S., Naughton, B., Saxonov, S., Avey, L., Wocjicki, A., Pe'ers, I. and Mountain, J. (2010) 'Web-based, participant-driven studies yield novel genetic associations for common traits', *PLoS Genetics*, vol. 6, no. 6, article e1000993, doi:10.1371/journal.pgen.1000993

Frazzetto, G. (2009) 'Genetics of behaviour and psychiatric disorders: From the laboratory to society and back', *Current Science*, vol. 97, no. 11, pp. 1555–1563.

Genetics and Public Policy Center (2010) 'DTC genetic testing companies', 28 May, available at https://web.archive.org/web/20100821110423/http://www.dnapolicy.org/resources/AlphabetizedDTCGeneticTestingCompanies.pdf (accessed 7 February 2011).

GenomeWeb (2012) 'Integrated analysis defines potentially predictive schizophrenia risk genes', *GenomeWeb News*, 15 May, available at www.genomeweb.com/integrated-analysis-defines-potentially-predictive-schizophrenia-risk-genes (accessed 2 December 2015).

George, D., Whitehouse, P. and Ballenger, J. (2011) 'The evolving classification of dementia: Placing the DSM-V in a meaningful historical and cultural context and pondering the future of "Alzheimer's"', *Culture, Medicine and Psychiatry*, vol. 35, pp. 417–435.

Groves, C. and Tutton, R. (2013) 'Walking the tightrope: Expectations and standards in personal genomics', *BioSocieties*, vol. 8, pp. 181–204.

Harvey, A. (2010) 'Genetic risks and healthy choices: Creating citizen-consumers of genetic services through empowerment and facilitation', *Sociology of Health and Illness*, vol. 32, no. 3, pp. 365–381.

Hedgecoe, A. (2001) 'Schizophrenia and the narrative of enlightened geneticization', *Social Studies of Science*, vol. 31, no. 6, pp. 875–911.

Hedgecoe, A. (2006) 'Pharmacogenetics as alien science: Alzheimer's Disease, core sets and expectations', *Social Studies of Science*, vol. 36, no. 5, pp. 723–752.

Hine, C. (2006) 'Databases as scientific instruments and their role in the ordering of scientific work', *Social Studies of Science*, vol. 36, no. 2, pp. 269–298.

Hudson, K., Javitt, G., Burke, W. and Byers, P. with the ASHG Social Issues Committee (2007) 'ASHG statement on direct-to-consumer genetic testing in the United States', *American Journal of Human Genetics*, vol. 81, pp. 635– 637.

Insel, T. R. and Wang, P. S. (2010) 'Rethinking mental illness', *JAMA: Journal of the American Medical Association*, vol. 303, no. 19, pp. 1970–1971.

Kawa, S. and Giordano, J. (2012) 'A brief historicity of the Diagnostic and Statistical Manual of Mental Disorders: Issues and implications for the future of psychiatric canon and practice', *Philosophy, Ethics and Humanities in Medicine*, vol. 7, no. 2, available at www.peh-med.com/content/7/1/2 (accessed 15 September 2015).

Latour, B. (1987) *Science in action: How to follow scientists and engineers through society*, Cambridge, MA: Harvard University Press.

Leonelli, S. (2012) When humans are the exception: cross-species databases at the interface of biological and clinical research. *Social Studies of Science* vol. 42, no. 2, pp. 214–236.

Lerner-Ellis, J. P., Ellis, D. J. and Green, R. (2013) 'Direct-to-consumer genetic testing: what's the prognosis?', *GeneWatch*, available at www.councilforresponsiblegenetics.org/genewatch/GeneWatchPage.aspx?pageId=277 (accessed 15 August 2013).

Lewontin, R. (1991) *Biology as ideology: The doctrine of DNA*. New York: HarperPerennial.

Lightman, B. (2011) 'Victorian periodicals, evolution, and public controversy', *Spontaneous Generations*, vol. 5, no. 1, pp. 5–11.

M'Charek, A. (2013) 'Beyond fact or fiction: On the materiality of race in practice', *Cultural Anthropology*, vol. 28, no.3, pp. 420–442, doi: 10.1111/cuan.12012.

MacKenzie, D. (1990) *Inventing accuracy. A historical sociology of nuclear missile guidance*, Cambridge, MA: MIT Press.

Maiti, S., Kumar, K. H. B. G., Castellani, C. A., O'Reilly, R. and Singh, S. M. (2011) 'Ontogenetic de novo copy number variations (CNVs) as a source of genetic individuality: Studies on two families with MZD twins for schizophrenia', *PLoS ONE*, vol. 6, no. 6, pp. 1–13.

Mitchell, P. B., Meiser, B., Wilde, A., Fullerton, J., Donald, J. Wilhelm, K. and Schofield, P. R. (2010) 'Predictive and diagnostic genetic testing in psychiatry', *Psychiatric Clinics of North America*, vol. 33, pp. 225–243.

Morrison, M. (2012) Promissory futures and possible pasts: The dynamics of contemporary expectations in regenerative medicine', *BioSocieties*, vol. 7, pp. 3–22.

National Society of Genetic Counselors (2010) 'Press release: Consumers should be mindful of DTC genetic testing: Don't bypass genetic counselors, medical geneticists or other healthcare providers', available at www.nsgc.org/Portals/0/Press%20 Releases/DTC_Press_Release_020410.pdf (accessed 15 September 2012).

Owen, M., McGuffin, P. and Gottesman, I. (2003) 'The future and post-genomic psychiatry, in P. McGuffin, M. Owen and I. Gottesman (eds), *Psychiatric genetics and genomics*, Oxford: Oxford University Press, pp. 445–460.

Parliamentary Office of Science and Technology (2012) *Consumer genetic testing: Postnote 407*, London: Houses of Parliament.

Persson, A. and Welin, S. (2008) *Contested technologies: Xenotransplantation and human embryonic stem cells*, Lund, Sweden: Nordic Academic Press.

Rabeharisoa, V. and Bourret, P. (2009) 'Staging and weighting evidence in biomedicine', *Social Studies of Science*, vol. 39, no. 5, pp. 691–715.

Schizophrenia Psychiatric Genome-Wide Association Study Consortium (2011) 'Genome-wide association study identifies five new schizophrenia loci', *Nature Genetics*, vol. 43, no. 10, pp. 969–976.

Shapin, S. and Schaffer, S. (1985) *Leviathan and the air pump: Hobbes, Boyle and the experimental life*, Princeton, NJ: Princeton University Press.

Siles, I. (2011) 'From online filter to web format: Articulating materiality and meaning in the early history of blogs', *Social Studies of Science*, vol. 41, no. 5, pp. 737–758.

Spandler, H. (2009) 'Spaces of scientific contention: A case study of a therapeutic community', *Health and Place*, vol. 15, pp. 672–678.

Suryanarayanan, S. and Kleinman, D. L. (2013) 'Be(e)coming experts: The controversy over insecticides in the honey bee colony collapse disorder', *Social Studies of Science*, vol. 42, no. 2, pp. 215–240.

Tienari, P., Wynne, L. C., Sorri, A., Lahti, I., Läksy, K., Moring, J., Naarala, M., Nieminen, P. and Wahlberg, K-E. (2004) 'Genotype-environment interaction in schizophrenia-spectrum disorder: Long-term follow-up study of Finnish adoptees', *British Journal of Psychiatry*, vol. 184, no. 3, pp. 216–222.

Trapp, D. (2010) 'Consumer genetic testing has little value, GAO report says', *American Medical News*, 2 August, www.amednews.com/article/20100802/government/ 308029944/7/.

Walsh, T., *et al.* (2008) 'Rare structural variants disrupt multiple genes in neurodevelopmental pathways in schizophrenia', *Science*, vol. 320, no. 5875, pp. 539–543.

Wouters, P., Beaulieu, A., Scharnhorst, A. and Wyatt, S. (eds) (2013) *Virtual knowledge: Experimenting in the humanities and the social sciences*, Cambridge, MA: MIT Press.

Wyatt, S., Harris, A., Adams, S. and Kelly, S. (2013) 'Illness online: Self-reported data and questions of trust in medical and social research', *Theory, Culture and Society*, vol. 30, no. 4, pp. 128–147.

Wyatt, S., Harris, A. and Kelly, S. (2016) 'Controversy goes online: Schizophrenia genetics on Wikipedia', *Science and Technology Studies*, vol. 29, no. 1, pp. 13–29.

Wynne, B. (1992) 'Misunderstood misunderstanding: Social identities and public uptake of science', *Public Understanding of Science*, vol. 1, no. 3, pp. 281–304.

Conclusion

CyberGenetic futures

Preventive measures

by Caoilinn Hughes

Today, I wanted to show you my heart.
You asked, 'You'd open your ribs like a book?'

Blood vessels broke on your cheeks and you shook.
I wanted to help you to see, label the troublesome parts.

'I regret the faults I passed on, but that's the Lord's unknowable way.
I've more stents now than prayers and they serve me just fine.'

Dad, I wanted to show you the organ I ordered online.
It's the colour of cider apple. It's complex as your ear. Tender as stingray.

You glanced at the jar stuck between us. The muscle it held was lightened.
The preservant was bloodstained like Reisling poured on the dregs of Syrah.

You can wear my old heart on your sleeve, I laughed. You said, 'A stigma?'
You sat there, heart bleating, until apples in some orchard had ripened.

'Preventive measures' dramatises how different generations feel responsibility for one another, and how they cope with and communicate about change. Developments in medicine and healthcare play a role in these changing relationships that can involve promise and hope, but also regret, fear and guilt. The rhythm of the poem, when read aloud, intensifies the tension between the father and child. The poem addresses some of the main themes of this book, about how knowledge of genetics and modern medicine can reconfigure time, space, identity and social relationships.

This book opened with a composite account of what it was to order a spit kit and to receive the results. We have returned to that imaginary user throughout the book in order to illustrate different aspects of the DTC genetic testing process. In the Introduction, one of us, Susan Kelly, shared her own experiences of being a customer of 23andMe, in an autoethnographic account that both informed and was informed by our analysis, prefiguring what we later referred to as 'autobiology'.

In this final chapter, we continue with these more experimental forms of writing, harking back to the radical reflexivity more common in STS in the late 1980s and early 1990s (see Woolgar, 1988). We present three (semi-)fictional accounts for how DTC genetic testing might develop. These illustrate some of the recurring themes in the book, about genetic and other forms of determinism, about the role of private companies in healthcare and medical research, about what genetic knowledge does for our sense of self, and our trust in ourselves and others, and the sometimes hidden, sometimes quite visible role of digital technologies in these processes.

We have deliberately chosen speculative fiction to reflect upon the role of future imaginaries in the emergence of techno-scientific phenomena. It is not only the poet who creates and imagines a future from current and promised science. Technological developments such as genetic testing grow from projections of what is possible in the future. They feed off and feed into public imaginations which can be expressed in many forms, and affect how we all imagine the future. The mental healthcare service users whom we interviewed were ambivalent about buying genetic tests online. They imagined genetics as solving problems with mental health treatment and stigma, but were wary of corporate interests and ownership in such a future. One of the participants whom we interviewed provided her own imagination of a future of genetic testing, further expressing ambivalence about the promises of this technology:

> I think there is sort of a 'brave new world' worry about genetics, that ... this is what any sane, rational person would want to do or should do, be tested and not have children if they find themselves to be a carrier of, I don't know... familial Mediterranean fever ... it risks a sort of slippery slope in which people feel under some sort of obligation to do the decent thing.
>
> I've thought a lot about how we walk into our futures backwards, how we're made to walk into our future backwards, so we are only looking back at the things we've experienced, we don't know what is behind us and we have to walk backwards. Those people who know some things, who've been able to turn round and look in the other direction are, it's almost got a sort of ring of Greek mythology to it. It's something of a curse ... that, for example, lot of gain, virtually no loss [in testing for] coeliac disease, is definitely helpful. Alzheimer disease, or multi-infarct dementia [testing for these could be 'something of a curse'] ... that is turning round and walking the wrong way into your future., so I want to walk into mine backwards.

Our own imaginations as researchers are visible in the project proposal that Susan and Sally wrote in order to obtain funding for this research. The DTC genetic testing field was a remarkably different landscape in mid-2010, than what had emerged by the time of writing this book, five years later, with developments we could have hardly predicted. Many of the psychiatric genetic testing companies we first identified for example, were no longer selling their tests. 23andMe had more fully expanded into research, patents and publications. Personalised medicine, whole genome sequencing, and emerging forms of consent for participation in biomedical research have become active fields of debate that engage the themes we have identified throughout this book. The fields of genetics and digital technologies are rife with 'promissory' futures and hopeful presentations (Morrison, 2012; Tutton, 2011), and have come together in ways that resonate with big societal themes, themes we explore in this book.

By presenting three further imaginary futures in three fictions we offer a playful glimpse into what might be possible. In doing so, we intend to escape, as Nowotny (2008) encourages us to do, the usual polarities of dystopian and utopian futures, by exploring the underlying ambivalence that we found pervades techno-scientific phenomena such as DTC genetic testing, and which we see in many other engagements with current healthcare technologies. The stories are presented here in chronological order, although as a reader you may wish to pick and choose, and create your own timeline, at the same time imagining your own possibilities for walking backwards or forwards into the future.

Letters from the lake

Hermance, Switzerland
To Prof Stephen Whitefield, Devon, England

2 April 2015

You will be happy to hear that I/we have arrived and settled into our rooms, and no disaster has befallen us at the beginning of this period of work. I want to assure you that we could not be in a better place for accomplishing the task we have set out, although I do regret that you aren't here with me.

So here I am on the shores of Lake Lamond, near where Mary Shelley wrote Frankenstein, just outside Geneva. The weather is better for us than it was for them, although I hope we'll also be productive. At least we won't be trying to scare each other! I thought instead that I would write letters to you (very old-fashioned and non-digital!) to keep track of my experiences here.

Of course, I am re-reading Frankenstein, and thinking about the work we are embarking upon. Reading it again fills me with the excitement of discovery! And causes me to reflect on how different it was to approach science, knowledge production, in those days.

Mary Shelley wrote: 'this story was begun in the majestic region where the scene is principally laid, and in society which cannot cease to be regretted. I passed the summer of 1816 in the environs of Geneva.'

We are lucky enough to be working in similarly majestic environs, although it keeps me away from you and home. Thank you for letting me go! It is comforting nonetheless to know that you can keep track of me, with that app I left on your computer. You can track my sleep, my exercise, my nutrition. My heart beat! It is a bit like my data double being there keeping you company! That's a bit creepy. But also fun! I never thought I would so much enjoy keeping track of myself in this way. I suppose it makes me feel responsible and healthy, as well as a bit close to you. It is interesting to think that you are not the only other person I am sharing my data, my self! with. These various devices do the communication for me to these distant others, and I am not directly involved. I realise that I do not know how these communications occur, they are not transparent to me, but surely in order to be in charge of myself in this way, I must trust it. I am contributing part of myself to something greater! (now I sound political).

Anyway, back to Frankenstein. It is interesting to think about how differently people wrote to each other and expressed their emotions, and I imagine experienced the world, than do you and I. We are so used to communicating by email and text, this tangible paper and ink-based communication seems strange. I feel that Victor Frankenstein is very much, as a particular kind of person communicating particular feelings via a particular modality, part of the ecosystem of science of his time. As am I, I suppose. Interesting to think about, to entertain my mind while away from you.

Your loving wife,
Susan

Hermance, Switzerland
To Prof Stephen Whitefield, Devon, England

5 April 2015

How quickly time passes here, aware as we are of the size of the task before us! The weather is distractingly lovely, although a chilly breeze blows across the lake forcing us to keep jumpers and jackets to hand. We have made progress, having outlined the work and assigned tasks to ourselves. The themes of our work are emerging.

A slight glitch has occurred, however. As you can tell from my data monitors, I had a wee accident and injured myself yesterday. I was taking a lovely walk on a country lane outside Hermance in the afternoon, watching the curious birds and paying no attention to the pavement beneath my feet, and fell directly into a pothole, spraining my ankle. It hurt so, I hope it heals quickly. According to my genetic test results, it should.

In spite of this, I remain excited about our work. And more often, I think about how I am participating in science, as I contribute these bits of myself to a larger effort to improve knowledge of human health. It is interesting to reflect that not that long ago, science was a solitary and broad endeavour; I must return to Victor Frankenstein again, and his excitement about 'natural philosophy'! He still had worlds to explore, and dreamed about places where his would be the first human footsteps! I have ill-kept roads to walk upon, and am highly specialised and in the company of many others.

I am increasingly plagued by questions of science, and of identity. Is the digital data I am 'creating' and sending out into the world 'me' in some fundamental sense, my given biology, and the results of my choices? What is it evidence of? And how is it of value? There is something incredibly poignant and sad about how Victor Frankenstein puts all of his vital energies into bestowing life onto a creature that is separate from him. Alienated. And sending it out into the world unwatched and unloved. I feel that I am beginning to understand this part of the story a bit better.

In any event, I remain your loving wife.

Susan

Hermance, Switzerland
To Prof Stephen Whitefield, Devon, England

20 April 2025

It was wonderful to see you. Thank you so much for making the journey here. I particularly enjoyed our train journey together through the mountains. Very refreshing as we get back to work. And to my reading! Of which you are by now most heartily sick. And we must bring this work to some kind of conclusion.

I have been thinking too much, and I can't help but wonder what 'freely partici-pate' means, especially when I wander between these parallel worlds of 'new' science, monster creation and 'genetics goes online.' In what sense, free? Do I contribute my data out of a sense of altruism, or curiosity, or fun, or interest in science? I wonder about such confusion of motives!

I am fixated on the image of 'the monster' who was not, when created, a monster but a thing of wonder, the manifestation of ego and hope and promise, nonetheless let out in the world, its behaviour and feelings unintended. Kind of like genetics let out of the clinic, or that blob of spit that starts it all off! Alienated. And thinking of the kind of person who would do this. And at the same time, of the kind of person who would not.

I feel that the work I am doing with my colleagues requires us to think hard about what is genetic information provided by tests, outside of the clinic where it is conventionally given meaning within the clinical setting and relationship. Is it a socio-technical artefact? And it may be useful to think, artefact of what? Not only of the specific technology that extracts DNA from spit in a spittoon, and sequences that DNA within particular parameters selected by the producer of the sequence, not only of the digital technologies that make sequencing and sharing possible, it is discursively made meaningful in its 'free' life outside the clinic, somewhat as the monster runs around outside Frankenstein's laboratory and meaning is made of him in various ways, meaning he is (evidently) hungry for.

I simply can't believe each time I read the story that this highly sensitive and intelligent young man abandoned his creation, a creature upon which he had bestowed life, to the world, without giving it meaning. In a sense, I see the rest of the book, post his abandonment of the creature, as a process of meaning making, and making meaning of himself and what he has done as well as of the creature. In a sense, the creature is a mirror of himself as creator. One the creator, the other the master! And this suggests that we look to the creators of genomic test products to understand better the nature of their creation. While, although they use the language of 'your genome' and 'you have a right to your information', it is no more my genome than the monster is 'himself', composed as he is of multiple body parts, but nonetheless, he is imbued with human subjectivity. I won't dwell on what it means to have a mind, and be a person, that is beyond my task here. But I am interested in what kinds of persons are made possible under different regimes of creation, of materially-shaped possibilities for being. I think that is a bit where Frankenstein leads me, the question of possibilities for being, and where being producers of knowledge fits into that question, their responsibility. And ours.

Do I believe I am my genes? Not really. So why do I feel that I am giving something of myself, and participating in a bigger project of 'health' than merely my own? I feel quite entangled in relationships I don't really understand. Perhaps I should come home now.

Your loving wife,
Susan

GenULuv announces entry to stock market

From our economics correspondent

26 August 2024

In one of the most hotly anticipated flotations in months, GenULuv announced today that it will join the stock exchange. GenULuv shook up the online dating market when it started operations on 14 February 2023. In its 18 months of operations, it has attracted over 250 million users worldwide, and claims that over 40 million conscious couplings have resulted from its novel way of bringing people together. GenULuv has a straightforward business model: it charges people to register for its compatibility matchings, and at the same time collects their genetic material.

The way it works is simple. Imagine you are looking for a long-term partner, or a potential parent to your future children. In the past, you would have had to go to parties or to work, or rely on friends or relatives to introduce you to their friends. In the middle of the twentieth century, you could have placed ads in 'newspapers' in which you specified your desires in as few words as possible, as in the pre-digital age you had to pay by the word. People used abbreviations to capture what they perceived to be their own qualities, or at least what they perceived others might be looking for. Archives of our print predecessor suggest that 'GSOH' was popular, but no one recalls what that actually means, and searches yield many alternatives. As the internet and social media took off at the turn of the century, so did online dating. In the early days of the internet, no one knew if you were a dog (another strange expression dating from the early internet years) but as time went on, it became very easy to check all sorts of details of potential friends and lovers. Before meeting them, you could check out their photos from the day they were born to their university graduation. At that time, many dating sites offered psychological matching, but there were risks with such methods as people were always trying to second guess what potential mates might be looking for, and people became very skilled in completing such questionnaires.

GenULuv exploited an important market opportunity when it started offering genetic tests as the basis for finding a partner, for the long or short term. Genes don't lie. For the basic service, you simply transfer the funds, send in a cheek swab, and wait for the suggested matches to arrive. The basic package includes menu suggestions for the bridal party, taking account of the food intolerances and salt/sweet preferences of the couple and their immediate genetic kin. There are extra packages which cost considerably more. For example, you could arrange for the guests at your wedding to find the best match among the other guests. Or you can indicate your preferences for your unborn children, to ensure you receive the right match. Another package includes mortgage advice, taking account of the longevity genes of both partners. There is also an option to link your GenULuv account with your GPS, to heighten the possibility of 'accidentally' meeting your future mate. Of course, this doesn't always work as your ideal mate may live on the other side of the world.

Initially, there was concern that this method of coupling would lead to massive unemployment among divorce lawyers. However, new opportunities for the legal profession have opened up. Earlier this year, there was a prominent case involving a couple who had met via GenULuv, a British man and a Sudanese woman. Since closing the Channel Tunnel and strengthening the sea defences in 2018, the British Government has strenuously worked to prevent entry of all non-British born people. However, given Article 16 of the Universal Declaration of Human Rights, and the fact that the woman could demonstrate her British genes (perhaps from a slave trader in the early eighteenth century), the couple successfully fought for their right to be together. The longer term legal implications remain unclear. Given the continued growth of the GenULuv database, and the ongoing research in compatibility, it may be that couples once considered perfect for one another, turn out to have a higher than average chance of conscious uncoupling, so the divorce lawyers are not yet looking for alternative work. And they are certainly considering who is liable.

There will always be people looking for love, but the real money is in the massive database the company has put together. Earlier this month, there were rumours that 23andMe was planning to buy GenULuv outright in order to combine the two biobanks. There have also been rumours that Privacy International will succeed in its attempts to block the trade in human genetic material. Prominent neuroscientists have contributed to the uncertainty as they question the scientific basis for genetic testing, drawing parallels with astrology and phrenology. Such rumours and controversy are fuelling the speculation over how the market will react when the company launches next month.

Online genetic testing: an archaeological assessment

Prepared for FUTURE Archaeology Ltd

26 June 2043

1. Introduction

In August 2041 Swedish data technicians unexpectedly stumbled across the partial and disarticulated digital genetic remains of 500,852 human individuals while dismantling a decommissioned server farm in Luleå, in the Arctic North. FUTURE Archaeology Ltd was commissioned to undertake further archaeological investigation of this remarkable discovery. Initial analysis revealed that the remains consisted of the online accounts of users of what was once called direct-to-consumer (DTC) genetic testing, an internet service used by those curious to learn more about the genetic basis of disease and ancestry.

The 2041 discovery has subsequently led to the unravelling of a global network of websites, blogs, videos, tweets and fora comments related to DTC genetic testing, and to connections with previously unexplained archaeological ruins in an Indian waste disposal site, of what we now know are 'spit kits' used in the testing process. This report outlines the main findings of the excavation work in Sweden and analysis of these related sites and objects.

2. The sites

Site A: The Luleå server farm in northern Sweden was an important data storage site for many online companies in Europe, intended for use between 2034 and 2043 AD. In 2041 the site was commissioned for early dismantling due to a series of electronic malfunctions in the cooling system, speculated to be related to unexpectedly warm Arctic temperatures in the summer of 2040 AD. The initial discoveries of user accounts were made during this dismantling, in Row 2.134, in warehouse AC612 of the server farm. Subsequent archaeological excavation in numerous servers around the world, particularly in the Silicon Valley, led to the later discoveries of the other online sites linked to these Luleå remains.

Site B: Since the Luleå discoveries in 2041 we have now connected several other previously unexplained artefacts to the online genetic testing phenomenon. In 2040 large quantities of plastic vessels of unknown origin were discovered by Indian waste archaeologists searching the site for remnants of iPads, iPhones and other disused objects in a vacuum waste processing plant in Kerala, India. The

Kerala waste disposal system is a major site for the treatment of medical waste generated by the city's hospitals and research centres. Archival documents show that this waste treatment plant serviced the Kerala Community hospital, which was commissioned in 2034 by several US-based genetic testing companies to perform analysis of spit samples submitted by their European customers. The plastic vessels were collected and stored by the Internet Museum in Kerala, for later analysis.

3. Main findings

The user accounts

The user accounts discovered in Luleå, of 500,852 individuals who had enrolled in direct-to-consumer genetic testing, yielded names, addresses, bank account numbers, results of genetic analysis, forum and blog comments, as well as answers provided by the users to health questionnaires. There was also evidence of connections between users, which seem to have occurred through a relationship finding application. It is unclear why this material was no longer password protected, nor if the individuals were aware of this amassed data. The results of genetic analysis displayed in user accounts, through pictures, diagrams and statistics, the predisposition that users had to diseases which are now very common in modern populations (such as heart disease), and others, which have changed classification (such as schizophrenia). Curiously, for each disease, several research articles on the once-used technique of genome-wide association testing were used as solid evidence of genetic association.

The connected websites

Further excavation of these user profiles revealed that they were part of a much denser DTC genetic testing network. Through hyperlink analysis and the Internet Archive, we found websites, fora, blogs, YouTube videos, photos, tweets and other social media related to the phenomena. It appears that at one stage there was a significant number of DTC genetic testing companies in operation, although several of these, particularly those testing for psychiatric illness, disappeared in the early days of the industry.

The spit kits

The vessels found in Kerala measured 5cm in length, and consisted of clear plastic tubing with a blue plastic cap lid and sticky label. Macroscopic analysis of the vessels as outlined by Mahammad *et al* (2039) revealed that they contained a mixture of human spit and other chemical agents. Indian archaeologists had connected the objects to spittoons used in 1900–1918 AD by those with tuberculosis to collect spit. We can now confirm that the Kerala disposal site objects are indeed also spittoons. We conducted further analysis on these items using virtual ethnographic analogy methods outlined by Xiang *et al.* (2038) and traced them back to an online genetic testing company which used these objects to collect spit for genetic analysis. Using archival video footage from YouTube, we have evidence of how these spittoons were used by the genetic testers, often in bedrooms or dining rooms.

4. Discussion

Analysed together, these digital and material fragments seem to document a small but once lively activity called direct-to-consumer genetic testing, which at its peak, in 2015, involved over one million users. Genetic testers seemed not only to find out about their genetic make-up but were also able to contact relatives, purchase musical scores based on their DNA, and engage in research projects.

Through the genetic test findings we could trace users who had engaged with this service as far back as 2007, with tests dating until 2017. The geographical distribution of users appears to be predominantly in the US until 2014, when numbers from the US dropped off dramatically, and we see users engaging the service from the UK and Canada.

While these numbers grew somewhat steadily over the years, in 2017 it appears that the sites were completely abandoned. We still have no evidence as to why this occurred and no singular explanation is universally accepted. There is speculation that the intended implementation of global medical device regulation laws may have prompted the collapse of this community. Others suggest that microbiome testing may have displaced genetic testing. The most popular theory, which we agree with, is that the genetic testing sites were only intended to exist temporarily, in order to build a database of material with which scientists could conduct commercially viable research for years to come.

5. Conclusion

The analysis of the Luleå findings, in conjunction with further internet archival analysis and analysis of the Kerala vessels, have revealed the remains of a small but once lively online genetic testing industry and to some extent, online community. The reasons for the abrupt end to online activities are inconclusive, although there is speculation that the users were part of a larger database-generating exercise. These findings have relevance for other internet archaeological excavations of once active and now dismantled communities from the same era, such as World of Warcraft gamers, mummy bloggers and self-trackers.

Acknowledgements

The authors would like to thank the Historic Swedish Internet Archaeology Service and the Kerala Internet Museum for their assistance with this report.

References

Mahammad, A. *et al.* (2039) *Contemporary approaches to macroscopic analysis*, Cambridge, UK: Cambridge Online Manuals to Archaeology.

Xiang, C. *et al.* (2038) 'New uses of ethnographic analogy in archaeology', *Archaeological Dialogues*, vol. 24, no. 3, pp. 192–202.

* * *

Each of these fictions imagines the main themes we have been threading throughout this book in different ways. Susan's letters to her husband deliberately evoke Mary Shelley's *Frankenstein* (1818/1994). They continue the autobiographical account she presented in the Introduction, but now in fictional form. It is about the creation of the 'dispersed biosubject' (see below) in the form of a letter written to her husband, modelled closely on the letters from Dr Frankenstein to his sister. Susan uses the language of empowerment and self-discovery, the new Prometheus via personalised medicine and participation in science, the optimised genetic self. She reflects on the virtues of science, and how science has changed, invoking Victor Frankenstein's sometimes naïve perspective. But just as Frankenstein had to deal with what he had created, Susan is also concerned about the treacheries of genetic knowledge, and the virtues of collective data sharing. Mary Shelley examined the notion of the individual scientist, labouring away in isolation, seeking the glory of discovery through the attainment of knowledge, and Susan is exploring how an autodidact negotiates the contemporary techno-scientific landscape. In this contemporary story, the internet offers a Northwest Passage means of discovery, simultaneously full of fear and dread and enabling rapid transit to distant shores of knowledge/promise.

Sally moves a bit further into the imagined future in order to explore another way in which DTC genetic testing might enter everyday life. Adopting a more satirical tone in an online newspaper article from the year 2024, she highlights the ways in which technoscience is intricately interwoven with financial markets and economic concerns. As we learn more about the fictional company joining the stock exchange (which has precedents in tailored online dating for example), the potential consequences of genetics going online are taken to a further, more mundane level, where we no longer find 'new' media meeting 'new' genetics, but rather that the technologies have become integrated unquestioningly into everyday practices and life events. Dating and wedding planning are taken to new heights, from tracking down mates, to tailored menus and future children; migration is reconfigured; coupling takes on a new form. Sally's account questions what data amassed in such enterprises mean in terms of ownership of genetic goods, about the continuing controversies about how science proceeds, with science as a challenge to political, economic, and social structures.

Anna projects further into the future, and finds traces of current practices surviving in digital and material form. Relating to our theme of trust, we find that promises made regarding how personal digital data will be stored and managed appear to have been as ephemeral as, in hindsight, were the genetic discovery activities for which they were generated. What has happened to the aggregation of digital traces amassed by companies and other actors in the name of future benefit? What has happened to promises of privacy protection? What of the long-term curation of digital traces? Under whose responsibility does this curation fall? Anna's account reminds us of the temporality of these enthusiasms, promises, arguments and contracts, including the temporality of determinisms we have found threaded throughout this work. She reminds us also of the largely invisible infrastructure of the digital world perhaps not equally invisible to all of those who engage with genetics online, from customers, to healthcare professionals, to companies amassing large databases. In this book, we have attended to the mundane practices such as spitting that are part of the complex of objects, discourses and practices that constitute the DTC genetic testing industry. These appear again as artefacts such as spittoons, the meaning and use of which can only be guessed at, far in the future. Anna reminds us that these elements have relationships with disparate persons and activities across the world, and that the digital is not merely virtual but connects in interesting ways with materiality. The temporality of our own knowledge production practices and methods is further highlighted.

We are brought back to one of our original questions, what happens when genetics goes online? We have examined new spatial-temporal arrangements made possible by this intersection of technologies and science, and found not only the importance of temporality, but emerging forms of participation, of being a 'user' of technology, of challenges to trust, and emerging representations of science. We have reflected on how we can study these phenomena that are constantly in flux.

The disparately located forms of work, agency and engagement we found initially with DTC genetic testing, beginning with spitting and on through receiving interpretations of personal genomic data, looser engagements with healthcare professionals and new interactions with private companies, has caused us to reflect on the nature of medical and scientific authority, on different ideas about participation and engagement in science, and on different forms of trust that are emerging in this 'brave new world' of cybergenetics.

The access that genetic testing consumers have to their 'raw data' certainly opens up new ways of engaging with the scientific literature, scientists, and the practice of science. The companies active in this field offer their customers access to their individual raw data. They provide further dynamic features built into the internet infrastructure, where the website becomes the face of the product, with layers of product engagement that were not previously possible. Websites are emerging where users can engage with their genetic data in increasingly creative ways, creating their own phenotypes and other research categories, encouraged to start their own research projects.

We have reflected on emerging 'users', whom we have sometimes also characterised as consumers, patients, research participants, citizen scientists and sources of data. We could capture this hybrid as an emerging 'dispersed biosubject', noting that beyond what we regard as rather superficial digital traces in how science is done ('big data'), there are changes in what it means to 'be' data, to know and to share one's biology, and the relations of trust that entails. We have noted that the normative framing of subject participation is shifting, a shifting of ethos from communities of science production to ones of participation. The notion of the 'dispersed biosubject' is meant as an extension of the notion of new forms of being described by Rose and Novas as 'biological citizenship': 'A new kind of citizenship is taking shape in the age of biomedicine, biotechnology and genomics' (Rose and Novas, 2005: 439). The dispersed biosubject refers to the subject taking shape in the age of biomedicine, digital technologies and genomics, the biosubject who is data, with gift obligations to variously situated others associated with that 'ownership', with possibilities stretched across time and space by digital communication. The biosubject is shaped by emerging normativities closely connected to personalised medicine, to citizen science, to self-tracking, themes we have explored. These biosubjects, as mentioned above, also have agency to create their own autobiologies, and to engage with the internet and with genetics in ways that may reinforce or resist the deterministic discourses accompanying both. Thus 'dispersed biosubjects' may well affect how cyberGenetics unfolds in the future.

References

Morrison, M. (2012) 'Promissory futures and possible pasts: The dynamics of contemporary expectations in regenerative medicine', *Biosocieties*, vol. 7, pp. 3–22.

Nowotny, H. (2008) *Insatiable curiosity: Innovation in a fragile future*, Cambridge, MA: MIT Press.

Rose, N. and Novas, C. (2005) 'Biological citizenship', in A. Ong and S. J. Collier (eds), *Global assemblages: Technology, politics and ethics as anthropological problems*, Oxford: Blackwell, pp. 439–463.

Shelley, M. W. (1818/1994) *Frankenstein, or, The modern Prometheus: The 1818 text*, ed. M. Butler, Oxford: Oxford University Press.

Tutton, R. (2011) 'Promising pessimism: Reading the futures to be avoided in biotech', *Social Studies of Science*, vol. 41, no. 3, pp. 411–429.

Woolgar, S. (ed.) (1988) *Radical reflexivity: New frontiers in the sociology of knowledge*, London: Sage.

Appendix A

New media, new genetics, new methods

Studying emergent phenomena is exciting, but also sometimes a bit unsettling. As we explained in Chapter 1, one risk is that simply by paying such close attention to the fascinating phenomenon of direct-to-consumer genetic testing, we contribute to its stabilisation and legitimacy. Similar anxieties apply to the internet generally and social media more specifically – that by studying them, we are also contributing to the realisation of the claims surrounding their transformative impacts, good or bad. There are also risks facing social scientists who may not be entirely sure of how to study novel social practices. The internet has opened up new possibilities for people to find and share information about their health, and for altering spatial–temporal arrangements between patients, healthcare professionals and private companies offering healthcare services. At the same time, the internet opens up possibilities for social scientists who study such people and phenomena, and who are interested in how this new medium affects the provision of healthcare services, including testing. Just as new instruments enable natural scientists to observe previously unseen phenomena, new media can also change the ways in which social scientists go about their work. This is particularly important as new media affect the abilities social scientists have to communicate about their work, not only among themselves, but also with their multiple audiences. As such, new media potentially intensify the speed at which ideas circulate.

In doing the research on which this book is based, we confronted a number of methodological and concomitant ethical choices. In this appendix, we discuss the choices we made. As such, we are behaving as responsible researchers, and providing further details for those readers who are interested in how we came to the conclusions presented earlier. But we also want to reflect on what digital media mean for social science research about health, illness, medicine and care. This is not a 'how to' guide for doing research about direct-to-consumer genetic testing, nor for any other similar phenomena that get stretched across time and place, with the potential for transforming not only social relations but also people's relationships with their own bodies. As Giddens (1976/1993) warned his readers in the preface to *New Rules of Sociological Method*, we are not offering a prescriptive set of rules. Instead we are proposing a set of considerations for those social scientists who recognise that the language and tools available to us as researchers are themselves changing, and they affect how we come to know and understand our objects of analysis. We have summarised the key principles guiding our approach to research in Box A.1.

Box A.1 Seven principles for doing research about emergent techno-scientific phenomena

We warned the reader above not to expect to find easy-to-follow guidelines about how to do research on emerging techno-scientific phenomena that take place in the world, a world that now encompasses both digital and analogue spaces. Nonetheless, we would like to put forward seven principles, based on our own experiences of doing research about DTC genetic testing. These principles may be useful for studying other phenomena that are heralded as transformative. The principles are not intended to be prescriptive, and we accept no responsibility for the results.

1   Keep notes about what you did, and keep screenshots or other evidence of what you found online. The digital world changes quickly, and you will not remember and may not be able to find material again, next year or even next month.
2   Take the phenomenon seriously. Understand what it is in its own terms. In our case, this meant not only genetic testing, but also the technical affordances of the online spaces we examined.
3   Remember that claims about transformations are not the same as transformations. Again, take the phenomenon seriously. One way to do this is to look at the mundane, everyday practices that are needed to make the phenomenon work in the world, even if it is as mundane as spitting. Consider all of the different people, groups, objects, protocols, assumptions that are needed to make the phenomenon work.
4   Think carefully about your methods, and be prepared to experiment with methods you have not previously used. Consider how your chosen methods contribute to the visibility and invisibility of people, objects and ideas.
5   Do no harm – neither to yourself nor to those about whom you are doing research. However, bear in mind that not all social groups are equal, and sometimes it is acceptable and even responsible to make normative judgements about the activities of powerful political and economic actors.
6   Be reflexive about your position as a social researcher. Remember that ideas about the socio-technical world are constantly circulating within and between those being researched, those doing the research, and those commenting on both, such as journalists and policy makers.
7   Dare to be creative. Sometimes visual or textual images can be more revealing. Experiment with alternative voices and forms of re-presentation.

Before discussing the specific methods we used to gather and analyse the material presented in earlier chapters, we first reflect on some of our own mundane methods, and the indispensability of digital technologies in the collaboration between the three of us, as authors of this book. In this way, we do recognise the enormous power of digital technologies, and the ways in which many aspects of academic practice are considerably easier than they were a generation ago. The availability of the internet facilitated our work enormously. During most of the time we worked on this book, we were located in Amsterdam, Calgary, Exeter and Maastricht (and rarely were more than two of us co-located), and for shorter periods of time at various conference and holiday destinations in Australia, Canada, the US and Europe. Digital technologies were central to our communication, and to our ability to prepare and share texts, using those now taken-for-granted applications of email, word processing, Skype and Dropbox. We also used the digital platforms available to many people living in Europe, and certainly to those working in universities, to identify and download literature and other sources, such as company registries. Digital methods are not only about high performance computing and computational techniques. They also encompass the everyday work of researchers in sometimes very mundane ways.

In the remainder of this appendix we reflect on our methods, first explaining how we gathered and analysed the material in each of the preceding chapters. We then reflect on ethics, ontology and epistemology, three themes that are of perennial concern to social scientists. In other words, we examine the ethics of doing research involving the online world, the ways in which methods bring objects of research (focusing on users) into being, and the researcher health warnings which should accompany all forays into digital methods about their epistemological implications.

Methodological choices made in preparation of this book

This section provides a chapter-by-chapter guide to how we collected data. As we conducted interviews with people in the UK, we needed to apply for ethical approval at the University of Exeter, where Harris and Kelly were based at the time. We obtained ethics approval from the College of Social Sciences and International Studies, University of Exeter on 31 May 2012 to conduct interviews with potential users of genetic tests, as well as an exemption from requiring approval for the internet research. In the Netherlands, it was not necessary to apply for ethical approval, neither at the time we applied for funding nor when we conducted the research. The Netherlands has had a relatively lax ethical regime for social science research, especially compared to what operates in Australia, Canada and the US. This is changing since the discovery of the spectacular research fraud committed by Diederik Stapel, a psychologist at Tilburg University (KNAW, 2013). We reflect more fully on the ethical implications of our choices later in this appendix.

Chapter 2: Users

Chapter 2 draws on interviews with users of mental health services, celebrity autobiography and videos found on YouTube made by users of genetic testing services. In February 2012, we queried the YouTube database for English-language videos uploaded by users of genetic testing services in a list of companies compiled by the Genetics and Public Policy Center (2010), including only those which concerned genetic testing for illness and traits. We found 20 videos in total, all uploaded by 23andMe, a company which actively engages with social media as an important aspect of its business profile, and a key actor throughout the book. In selecting videos we excluded explicitly promotional videos such as those posted by companies themselves; however, the delineation between promotional and non-promotional videos is not always clear.

The 20 videos in our sample broadly fit into three categories or genres: unboxing/spitting videos, logging into results, and retrospective descriptive accounts. In the 'unboxing/spitting' videos, people film themselves opening the 23andMe spit kit package and filling the tube with saliva. In the 'logging into results' videos, users share their results, and their interpretation of them. In the 'descriptive' videos, users describe either the process of taking the test, or the experience of reading their results. (Two of these videos also contained small sections of spitting footage.) Because we were interested in the performance of biological practice and the narrative interpretation of results we focused predominantly on the unboxing/spitting videos and the logging in videos.

Our unit of analysis was the posted video (visuals, speech and other sounds), including surrounding online content, such as other YouTube videos, hyperlinks and comments. We treated the videos as public texts, rather than as interactions with individuals. The ethical implications of this choice are discussed below. The YouTube material was analysed using thematic narrative analysis. As a guiding framework, we drew upon the work of Gubrium and Holstein (1998) who emphasise the context of a story's production. Gubrium and Holstein are interested in the conditions of storytelling, and its effects, considering the story process within the circumstances in which it unfolds, rather than viewing storytelling as an unmediated account of experience. They emphasise the social organisation and interactional dynamics of narratives. In this vein, we analysed the context for these stories, also keeping in mind the ways in which scholars in science and technology studies have problematised the notion of context, considering it not as something 'out there', 'to be found and explicated' (Asdal and Moser, 2012: 300), but rather as a process, imbued with materiality, by which a text, and its content and subject matter, is made (Asdal and Moser, 2012). We considered the material conditions of storytelling (bedrooms, computer hardware, spit kits, bedspreads, posters), texts (speech, computer software, the video image, hyperlinks), and issues (genetic testing available to the public, ambiguous states of illness), and the ways in which these are woven together in the story. We examined editing, both of the story being told and of the video, and performativity, examining how the storytellers position themselves in relation to the audience and other narratives.

We explored the embodied aspects of storytelling (facial expression, gestures, salivating, typing), intertextual components such as different mediums and platforms used and referred to, as well as how words, ideas and plots were drawn from other narratives. We considered these aspects in the context of the emerging market for DTC genetic testing, drawing upon our broader research in this area. Even though this material appears early in this book, it was done towards the end of our project.

We had identified genetic testing for psychiatric disorders as particularly challenging as the science is controversial even though some DTC genetic tests were on the market, raising the stakes concerning the industry. In order to better understand how these developments were viewed by persons living with mental illness, either with a diagnosis or as a carer, we undertook a series of in-depth, semi-structured interviews with people from these categories. As mentioned above, we obtained ethical approval from the University of Exeter to conduct these interviews. We then met with group of 'lay' people who are involved in research in Exeter through an organisation called PenPIG (Peninsula Patient Interest Group) on 29 March 2012. (More information about the group can be found here: http://clahrc-peninsula.nihr.ac.uk/meet-penpig.) We presented the project and our findings to date, showing websites of DTC companies and discussing the science as well as we could, and asked the group what they found interesting, and what kinds of things we should explore in our interviews. This meeting shaped the questions in our interview guide, together with the overarching research questions of the project. We recruited interview participants primarily through a local organisation, Be Involved Devon. Most participants were living with a diagnosis of mental disorder. We were able to interview only six people, despite a range of efforts to recruit participants. Face-to-face interviews were conducted by Susan Kelly, on the premises of the University of Exeter and took place from July to October 2012. The interviews were digitally recorded and transcribed, and analysed in terms of the themes that have emerged from our research. The interview participants were generally sceptical about the DTC industry and the science, although there was some view that at least some tests might have utility.

Chapter 3: Genetic counselling

For our analysis of the role of genetic counselling in DTC genetic testing, we compiled a list of company websites offering genetic testing services to consumers after consulting published literature (e.g. Hennen, Sauter and Van Den Cruyce, 2010), and a list of companies compiled by the Genetics and Public Policy Center (2010). This was done in December 2010, and was supplemented with online searches using various search engines (Google, Yahoo, Bing and Ask), by entering terms such as 'genetic testing' and 'direct to consumer genetic test'; and TouchGraph, a web link visualisation tool, by typing in the term 'genetic testing'. It is important to use multiple search engines, not only because users themselves have a choice but also because different search engines use different techniques to produce the results presented to users. The combined search generated a total of 52 websites. In January 2011, we analysed the content of these websites to delineate which companies explicitly offered genetic testing for mental health conditions as this was the initial focus of our research. Twenty companies were identified as meeting these criteria, which offered a diverse range of genetic testing services. Although the focus on companies selling tests for mental health conditions has had an influence on the kinds of companies in our sample, the 20 companies on our list included the most prominent, discussed and utilised companies in the market. These sites were then further analysed to obtain a list of those companies which also offered genetic counselling. The sites were entered into the Wayback Machine program, a website which provides archived webpages (see https://archive.org/web/web.php), to find previous versions of websites for each company in order to examine the history of counselling provision within the companies. In searching the internet to find companies selling genetic tests, other websites were also identified which related to DTC genetic testing and genetic counselling. A Google search was also performed to find forums, blogs and other sites where DTC genetic testing and genetic counselling were discussed. Our intent with this approach was to obtain as full a picture as possible of the online representations of genetic counselling in association with DTC genetic testing. Because the research did not include human subjects, the University of Exeter ethics committee (see also above) confirmed that the research was exempt from review.

Data collection yielded six DTC genetic testing websites offering genetic counselling either internally (by company employees) or by a third party; three blogs administered by DTC genetic companies which discussed genetic counselling services; four blogs discussing genetic counselling and DTC genetic testing, which were not administered by DTC genetic testing companies; and one interview which was available online with a genetic counsellor who discussed DTC genetic testing.

We archived all web material using WebCite (www.webcitation.org) and transferred written text to tables for ease of analysis. We performed discourse analysis of all material. Discourses were considered online texts in the form of the words, images and hyperlinks on company websites, whose combined meaning extends beyond the text itself (Denzin and Lincoln, 2011). We were concerned with the companies' accounts of genetic counselling practice and thus studied representations of genetic counsellors' roles within the industry. Discourse analysis drew upon a social constructionist epistemology which recognises that knowledge is situated and that language and discourse have a role in the way in which the genetic counselling profession is conceptualised (Hall, 1997). This strategy was appropriate considering our interest in how genetic counselling is represented in discourses online, recognising that our interpretation of these texts is only one of a number of possible readings. Analysis involved detailed and repeated readings of the texts, including visual material, looking for themes (Lupton, 1997). All three authors discussed these themes and further developed the analysis. We also analysed seven position statements by healthcare organisations in relation to DTC genetic testing and performed a literature review of research related to the DTC genetic testing industry and genetic counselling, genetic counselling more broadly, and telegenetics.

Chapter 4: Participation

The company 23andMe was the focus of our critique of how people were enrolled in genetic research. In July and August 2011, we collected the following material: company web pages; all versions of informed consent forms, privacy statements and terms of service downloaded from the website; rules for participation in community forums; press releases; blog posts (the 23andMe blog is called Spittoon); tweets; YouTube videos; patent applications; and research articles available on the internet published by 23andMe researchers, including two articles published in the open-access journal *PLoS Genetics* (Eriksson *et al.*, 2010; Do *et al.*, 2011) and one article published on the non-peer-reviewed website *Nature Precedings* (Tung *et al.*, 2011). To inform our analysis we also read forum posts on the 23andMe community pages. We then conducted discourse analysis, as described above. We did not have informed consent from users, thus we did not explicitly use forum material in our research. We return to this ethical issue below.

Chapter 5: Controversy

Our analysis focused on how the genetic basis for schizophrenia is presented and contested by companies selling genetic tests directly to the public. In October 2011, we updated the work we had done in late 2010 when we had focused on genetic counselling (see above). We looked for companies selling tests online for schizophrenia, again using various search engines (Google, Yahoo, Bing and Ask) and search terms such as 'schizophrenia & genetic testing'. We also consulted the August 2011 publication from the Genetics and Public Policy Center which listed genetic testing companies offering tests for disease groups, including mental illness. We identified three companies selling tests for schizophrenia: 23andMe, MapMyGene, and Lumigenix. Two companies making claims about, but not selling, genetic tests for schizophrenia were also identified: SureGene and DeCODEMe. Another company, Navigenics, specifically stated that it did not offer testing for schizophrenia because 'recent research into the genetic risk markers for this mental illness ha[ve] yielded inconsistent results'. Thus, already in the process of identifying DTC genetic testing companies, we observed contradictory views and activities related to testing for schizophrenia. From the selected websites, we focused on how the sites drew on scientific resources regarding schizophrenia genetic testing. We also followed schizophrenia genetics into the blogosphere, focusing on company-registered blogs administered by 23andMe (The Spittoon) and DeCODEMe (DeCODEYou). All blog material was collected in February 2011, and covered postings between March 2008 and February 2011. We surveyed all blog posts during this time (542 from 23andMe and 76 from

DeCODEYou) searching for entries relevant to schizophrenia genetics, and found five posts on the topic.

We collected web material from a range of platforms, looking at infrastructural details such as hyperlinks, which provide insight into how websites act as spaces for sharing and circulating scientific resources (Beaulieu, 2005; Rogers, 2013). We performed thematic analysis of all collected material including words, images and hyperlinks. Analysis involved detailed and repeated readings of the material, looking for themes (Lupton, 1997). When examining this material, we focused on how scientific resources were utilised. For example, we also read blog comments to examine further engagement with the scientific resources discussed in blog posts. (In another article, not discussed in this book, we examined how controversy around schizophrenia genetics was discussed on English-language Wikipedia 'talk pages'; see Wyatt, Harris and Kelly, 2016).

Finding material online: ethics of using self-reported data

In Chapter 4, we focused on how 23andMe makes use of both genetic and phenotypic data provided by people who pay to do so. Similar developments (though usually without asking people to pay) can be observed in the social sciences where the availability of vast quantities of online data generated by people as they shop, travel and visit websites and social media may, some claim, seem to obviate the need for traditional social science methods such as the survey, the interview or the focus group (Savage and Burrows, 2007). Social scientists have long grappled with the disjunction between what people say and what people do. The combination of utterances captured when people use social media and their traces (where they are, who they are communicating with and for how long, which websites they visit, and a multitude of other traces) when engaging in computer-mediated exchanges means that social scientists now have access both to what people say and what they do. This possibility for engaging in data-intensive methods raises epistemological and ontological questions, addressed below, but here we focus on the ethical ones.

Researchers are confronted with various ethical dilemmas when dealing with the vast quantities of data online, especially data generated by people going about their daily lives, either as traces of transactions and movements or as more-or-less considered reflections via social media. Are these data simply to be treated as any other publicly available information? If so, then appropriate citation and acknowledgement of sources solves many problems. For much information found online, that is indeed more than adequate. However, in informal settings, including many patient groups, such an approach would not meet the basic ethical principle, of protecting people, sometimes from themselves.

Debates around the privacy and anonymity of respondents (and researchers) have been well rehearsed (e.g. Ess and AoIR Ethics Working Committee, 2002; Ess, 2009; Wyatt, 2012). Problems arise because protecting the human subject is seen as the primary obligation of individual researchers, professional disciplinary associations and ethical review committees. It is assumed there is a simple, clear relationship between data found online and individuals in the real world. This is what Carusi (2008) calls 'thin' identity, and what Beaulieu and Estalella (2011) refer to as 'traceability'. Given that individuals may reveal a great deal of personal information online, researchers have to be concerned to protect the anonymity and privacy of research subjects. The danger facing social researchers and their respondents is that individuals could be easily identified and traced if, for example, their words, avatars, or nicknames are mentioned in academic texts. Even when attempts are made to anonymise individuals, other details (in combination with search engines with increasingly attuned algorithms) could more or less inadvertently enable their identification.

Individuals going about their everyday online lives are not obliged to be part of research. Even if they are voluntarily providing extensive details about their calorie intake, drug reactions or mental health status, it does not necessarily mean that this information is fair game for researchers. It is not always adequate for researchers to say this information is in the public domain. Nissenbaum (2010) discusses this in terms of 'contextual integrity' and draws attention to the expectations of privacy people may have in particular contexts, both online and offline. She highlights the right to privacy 'neither as a right to secrecy nor a right to control but a right to appropriate flow of personal information' (Nissenbaum, 2010: 127). Similarly, Bakardjieva and Feenberg (2000) point to the dangers of alienation arising from indiscriminate use of material found online, alienation experienced by people who have provided information in one context who may understandably not be happy to find it taken up in another. These concerns have become more acute with the rise of integrated data and more powerful search techniques, working precisely to cross contexts. Furthermore, healthcare practitioners, policy makers and researchers may sometimes have good reasons to integrate data about individuals from different domains in order, for example, to examine the relationship between income inequality and life expectancy, or to prevent adverse drug reactions.

Other scholars have pointed to the dangers associated with assuming an isomorphic relation between individuals and some of their online utterances, and argue for treating online material as forms of representation. By doing so, other ethical issues and responsibilities emerge. For White (2002), it is important to recognise the constructed nature of online material, so that researchers can challenge the abundance of hate speech that is easily found. She argues that by recognising the highly mediated and representational character of online material and by considering the ethical codes of literary studies or of art history and visual culture, different sorts of research questions can be addressed, opening up different forms of analysis. In a similar vein, Bishop (2009) bemoans the fact that a focus on the privacy of respondents makes it more difficult to consider the ethical obligations researchers may have to other actors and stakeholders.

Opening up the possibility that online data may be constructed by social actors for particular audiences in particular contexts, raises challenges, especially for medical researchers working within more realist research frameworks dominated by the RCT (randomised clinical trial), and for social scientists studying both everyday life and medical science. In many ways, these issues are neither new nor specific to web 2.0 and/or the health domain. Issues related to ethics, trust, representativeness, online identity, and so on have been raised since researchers began studying the web in the mid-1990s. But the web, social media and associated research opportunities continue to grow and change, which may lead to new issues, new iterations of old issues, or changes in the nature and scale of existing issues. This demands continued methodological reflexivity on the part of social science researchers, and continued attention to the relationships of trust with respondents, peers, funders and other stakeholders with whom they are involved.

As the 'participatory turn' broadens in scope and scale through digital self-reporting, researchers need to consider the implications of these mutual and fragile trust relationships for research and knowledge production practices. How self-reported data, constructed by subjectivities, becomes rhetorically empowered through various discursive practices on the web influences how we understand the social life of digital data. Our critical analysis of 23andMe and its practices in relation to the collection and use of self-reported data mediated by digital technologies therefore forced us to examine our own practices in using the data we found online, generated by people who, in contrast to 23andMe customers, may have no interest in supporting or being part of research. Of course, another important difference is that we do not seek to gain financial advantage even if we would like academic rewards in the form of research grants, peer-reviewed publications, citations and jobs. Digital research practices raise important questions for both medical and social science research: what is good research, or reliable and valid research? Is digitally mediated self-reported data any different from other types of self-reported data? What do we mean by a representative sample? How does the internet frame trust in data sharing between researchers and research participants, and among researchers? What constitutes ethical research practice? As data become more social and more mobile, do researchers need to re-consider how they interact with data and the people the data may or may not represent?

We have answered some of these questions in different ways. For example, we did not contact those who posted YouTube videos featuring spitting or opening their results (see Chapter 2) for their consent to analyse their videos. As discussed above, we did consider whether these people should be considered as autonomous individuals, creating texts for public consumption, or as social science research participants. In this instance, we chose for the former. Thus we treated the videos as public textual resources, similar to a television programme (Berry, 2004), and we analysed the audio-visual material of the video, and the surrounding online visual and written content. We came to this decision by considering the accessibility of the videos (no password required), and the ethos of the site which is to 'Broadcast Yourself' (part of the YouTube logo in its early, pre-Google days). While it could have been interesting to try to contact the YouTubers, especially in order to understand more about their engagement with DTC genetic testing (see also below), but for the purposes of this research, we were primarily interested in the texts themselves, and the context of these texts as video narratives shared with a public audience.

We came to a different decision regarding the material on some of the online fora of 23andMe. As we made clear in Chapter 1, Kelly did sign up to 23andMe, did pay for a spit kit and did receive her results, whereas Harris and Wyatt decided not to do so. Kelly's access to material as a 23andMe customer certainly informed her understanding of the phenomenon, and, indirectly, also that of Harris and Wyatt. But, as explained in Kelly's autoethnographic account in Chapter 1, we decided not to cite the material in forums that are behind the 23andMe paywall, and that are password-protected. We decided those comments were off limits to us as researchers, as those who had paid for 23andMe services did have a reasonable expectation of privacy, and were certainly not consenting to have their material used for research purposes (other than for those of 23andMe itself, of course – something which came as an unpleasant surprise for many of its customers; see Sterckx *et al.*, 2013).

Ontological issues of finding participants and defining 'users'

The ground-breaking work of Oudshoorn and Pinch (2005) brought users to the attention of science and technology studies (STS), and there has been much attention to how users are defined conceptually. But less attention has been paid to how users are defined methodologically. In this section, we discuss how research methods define users. Methods are ways of putting together actors and instruments, and it is widely acknowledged in STS that methods shape the nature of knowledge generated (although STS researchers have paid more attention to the methods of the scientists they study, and somewhat less to their own). Following from this we argue that different social science research methods bring particular kinds of users into being (Law, 2004). We contend that if we are going to think further about users, we need to think carefully about the methods we use to study them.

There are many terms in circulation to describe those people who look for health information, and make use of healthcare services. In countries such as the US, where healthcare is largely a private good, referring to such people as customers or consumers, has a certain logical consistency. In Europe and many other parts of the world, such language suggests a capitulation to neoliberal logics increasingly imposed on public healthcare regimes (Harris, Wathen and Wyatt, 2010). On a more positive note, the shift in language could be seen as liberating. Instead of mental health patients, people become users or clients of mental healthcare services. This could be seen as less stigmatising, though it does run the risk of denying a duty of care to people who may be suffering. As we argued in Chapters 2 and 4, DTC genetic testing companies themselves play with the category of 'user', addressing visitors to their sites variously as customers, patients and researchers in their participant-led research activities. In this section, we focus on how different methods (and sometimes also different terms) make different kinds of 'users' available for analysis. There have been numerous studies of the users of genetic testing (both those offered online and via more conventional routes) which have attempted to understand more about them using a range of research methodologies. In this section, we explore several of these methods.

Studying potential users

As is the case with many emergent technologies, researchers of DTC genetic tests have turned to potential users in order to study their perspectives, projections, fears, concerns and likely behaviours relating to the tests. These studies largely utilise hypothetical genetic testing scenarios or company advertisements, which are presented to a selected group of respondents. Examples from this body of research include a study of Facebook users (Lee and Crawley, 2009), question-naires distributed through the UK Twins Registry (Cherkas *et al.*, 2010) and an internet-based survey sent to a random sample of adult Americans (Neumann *et al.*, 2011). We also conducted our own interview study of potential users of DTC genetic tests in Devon (see above, and Chapter 2).

The users that come into being from these studies are labelled as 'informed consumers' or conversely as being 'misinformed'. These potential users are enrolled to engage in an exercise of the imagination, projecting themselves into the future, based on their experiences of the present and past. Many of these stud-ies aim to inform policy and other decisions about further developments and applications of the technology.

The limitations of such future-based scenario research however are acknowl-edged, with many commenting on a mismatch between intention and action. Many researchers using methods based around hypothetical futures often conclude that we need more research on '*actual* users', more research on what people do, rather than on what they say they would do in some imagined future. In the field of DTC genetic testing, one common way of doing this is to conduct an internet-based survey.

Surveys

There have been several articles published about DTC genetic testing users, using internet-based surveys, including one conducted by *Nature* (Maher, 2011) and another undertaken by a popular blog *Genomes Unzipped* (MacArthur, Morley and Jostins, 2010). These studies bring a health-seeking curious user into being. It may be a curious scientist in the case of *Nature*, or a curious amateur scientist, in the case of *Genomes Unzipped*. Using a telephone survey, Critchley and her colleagues (2015) found that Australians were less trusting of tests sold by commercial companies. These surveys presuppose a knowing, self-aware indi-vidual who can make clear risk assessments.

Internet-based surveys offer several advantages over traditional paper-based surveys. The geographical reach can be easily extended, and those who complete the surveys are also doing the work of data entry, saving the researcher consider-able effort in transcribing the results from paper to computer. The goal of survey studies is to achieve adequate sample sizes, in order to achieve statistical power.

Users become categorised and aggregated. Surveys are often critiqued as lending themselves to superficial answers to closed questions, decontextualising individuals from their broader networks. Some researchers of genetic testing, including ourselves, focus on individual accounts, collecting data through interviews, auto-ethnography or by studying public narratives.

Interviews with users

Interviews are largely celebrated by social researchers as providing access to everyday, ordinary, mundane accounts of users' engagements with technology, and are widely used within qualitative social sciences more generally. Especially for sensitive topics, interviews provide an opportunity for trust and empathy to develop between interviewer and respondent. However, for a relatively unusual practice, such as buying a genetic test via the internet, it can be difficult to find suitable respondents in the vicinity of the researcher. Of course, the internet could itself be the solution to this problem, and interviews are increasingly conducted via email (giving respondents time to consider their answers, though perhaps making it more difficult to establish rapport) or some form of teleconferencing. This may lead to those who are not comfortable with the technology being excluded from the potential pool of respondents, however.

One much cited paper about users of DTC genetic testing is McGowan, Fishman and Lambrix's (2010) sociological study of early adopters. They interviewed bloggers who had used the test, and concluded that these users were, as Oudshoorn and Pinch (2005) suggest, co-constructing the technologies in the making, and that in the process they were both optimistic and sceptical. To date, this remains one of the only published studies in which DTC genetic testers have been interviewed and is often quoted as the study reflecting user perspectives. The paper has a life of its own in the DTC genetic testing research community. (A few other papers on DTC users have been published, notably Vernez *et al.*, 2013, and Lee *et al.*, 2013.)

Autobiography, autoethnography, autobiology

Several academics have decided to act as their own informants and write autoethnographies about testing. In these accounts another kind of reflexive user comes into being. Autoethnographic reflexivity has long been central to the ethnographic enterprise, and it is now increasingly popular for social scientists to draw upon their own experience in their work. Autoethnographic accounts have been used to make sense of personal experiences with technologies. Henwood *et al.* (2001) argue that they provide a useful tool for capturing the ambiguity of many people's relationships with technology, and for examining the complexity of lived experiences which always involve complex interconnections of the categories commonly used by social scientists, such as gender, age and ethnicity. Such accounts are never unmediated, they are always constructions of the past through present concerns and interests.

Public narratives

For researchers who have not undertaken testing themselves, or do not have access to users to interview, there are an array of public accounts of genetic testing for analysis, what could be considered ready-made data. The accounts that have captured the attention of researchers have been written by celebrity scientists, journalists and other media figures. These analyses once again bring the celebrity user into focus, just as the image of the 'spitterati' described in Chapter 2. These users, similar to the autobiographical accounts of researchers, are reflexive and critical, often have privileged access to the technology and consider genetics as part of a broader repertoire of scientific understanding about life.

As we have seen in Chapter 2, the public now interested in genetic testing has broadened since the DTC tests were first launched. Not all public narratives are by professional journalists or celebrity geneticists. We became interested in these other public narratives, and that is why we looked on YouTube, as discussed above. We recognise that these videos, just like other autobiographical accounts, are mediated, constructed and created through the instruments and tools used to create them, whether they be webcams, computers, or publishing houses. They are also mediated via the ways in which we turn them into research material, capturing them with software programs, and coding the material into tables. All research methods and tools, whether they be survey instruments, audio-recorders or software programs, provide structure and order to the material available to researchers.

To conclude this section, we argue that the choice of methods brings different kinds of user communities into being. In the examples above, users were presumed to be health-seeking individuals (be they actual patients, pre-patients or patients-in-waiting), however our analysis of the websites demonstrated that the products are equally being marketed to doctors who need to order the tests. In such cases the user is as much the healthcare professional as any individual consumer or patient. By focusing on users, whether patients or professionals, we are not attentive to non-users, those who object to DTC genetic testing, or who decline to engage in research. The choice of methods may also render some groups invisible, with effects for the kind of knowledge produced. Having discussed the ontological implications of our methodological choices, we now turn to the epistemological considerations.

The internet is not the world: epistemological considerations of online research

In the section above about different methods for obtaining accounts from users of DTC genetic testing, we hinted at some of the relative advantages and disadvantages of using digital technologies to identify participants, and to conduct interviews and surveys. In this section, we focus on the affordances of digital technologies as both object and method. Our interrogation of the use of self-reported data by 23andMe gave us cause to reflect upon how we as social scientists conduct web-based research, and collect data from online environments. We have already addressed some of the ethical and ontological considerations, but in this section we turn our critical gaze onto the epistemological implications of the methodological choices of ourselves and others.

One of the most common mistakes, since the earliest days of the internet and research about the internet, is to assume that internet users are representative of the population as a whole. A variation of this is to assume that present users are 'early adopters', and are somehow typical of all future users. This is a version of both methodological and normative technological determinism, discussed in the opening chapter. As boyd and Crawford (2012) argue in their study of Twitter, users of a particular platform should not be taken to represent all people, just as choice of interview medium may exclude some potential respondents, as mentioned above.

Our analysis in late 2010 and early 2011 of the online DTC genetic testing landscape was limited by our focus on testing for mental disorders and by our use of English-language search terms. Nonetheless the sample our search generated did seem to be representative of the range of websites available at that time, at least for websites registered in English-speaking parts of the world, where DTC genetic testing was taking flight. Another limitation was our focus on the online representations of genetic counselling. Representations are important in shaping expectations and experiences, but an empirical examination of the actual work and practices performed by those employed in the DTC genetic testing industry could shed further light on this professional group.

Similarly, the research reported in Chapter 5 focused on the material that was publicly visible on the company websites. Thus we know very little about the demographic characteristics and motivations of those users writing blog comments, for example. We focused on company websites, but there are many other platforms and applications which need further research regarding their role in controversy, such as list-servs, fora and video-sharing sites. In the case of schizophrenia genetics for example, user fora could provide an important resource for understanding how patients and consumers share resources, as well as genetic data, phenotypic information and illness experience, these forms of knowledge engaging with, contradicting and replicating biomedical understandings and scientific research.

There are other examples of social science researchers who are concerned with health and medicine experimenting with digital methods. For example, Prior *et al.* (2011) used text mining techniques in order to analyse 54 interview transcripts. They checked for co-occurrences between terms, such as flu jab and side effects. Pajek, the social network software they used, calculates the coefficients for all co-occurrences and displays them diagrammatically. This has advantages, as it checks the veracity of the human analysis, and captures a lot of information very concisely. They do not indicate how helpful it was or whether it revealed things they might otherwise have missed, but they do point to some of the problems, including that the software could not distinguish between what the interviewer said and what the respondent said. That is not inherent to the software, but is more a question of providing appropriate data for the program to process. There are potentially many ways that text-mining and natural language processing could be used, for example to analyse self-help guides in order to understand changes over time, across countries, or the differences between material targeted at particular social groups or diseases. The results could be completely trivial, and just because one can use a computer it does not mean one should, but there is at least the possibility of conducting more experiments in order to understand what digital methods have to offer. There are many opportunities for representing research results, such as Robison's (2009) visualisation of how four different databases capture the research literature on autism.

Other possibilities include making greater use of hyperlink analysis, in order to see if online linkages bear any relationship to real world connections and relationships. This can be done at an organisational level, as we did in our use of TouchGraph to generate a list of groups involved in DTC genetic testing, but it can also be done at a conceptual level, to look for links between words and semantics that describe diseases, symptoms, and treatments.

Just as there are many online spaces that could be examined, there are also other research methods that could be explored, such as social network analyses, textual analysis of representations of ideal users by the websites, and studies of online testimonials and blog comments. Nonetheless, the selection of different methods used to study DTC genetic testing and the different objects (users or otherwise) generated by these methods together highlight the importance of choice of methods in the production of knowledge.

Future directions

Thinking about methods and platforms together means that we have to consider carefully the choices we make, and the ethical, ontological and epistemological consequences of these choices. The internet is an interesting object of research for medical sociology, STS and all social science concerned with health, healthcare and medicine. It is where many people, including patients and healthcare professionals, are finding and sharing data and information. It is part of the rich, multimedia landscape where people search for information to help them to understand their bodies, health, illness, experiences of doctors, hospitals, drugs and other treatments. Our approach to methods and the material means of their realisation aligns with those who consider the infrastructural details of the internet as a methodological tool to be important and worthy of analysis (Bowker *et al.*, 2010; Meyer and Schroeder, 2015; Ruppert, Law and Savage, 2013; Snee *et al.*, 2015; Wouters *et al.*, 2013).

In this book, we have attempted to demonstrate the importance of the digital as object, and we have also attempted to demonstrate its usefulness as a research tool for those social science researchers interested in health-related topics. Using 'digital methods' of whatever form does however demand new sorts of skills. Social science has often engaged in arguments about the relative virtues of qualitative and quantitative methods, and in the past social science has pioneered the use of new methods, such as interviews and focus groups. But there is now a danger that social scientists are being left behind by the corporate use of data-intensive and computational methods.

For example, on 13 April 2015, IBM announced that it is combining its cognitive computing technology, called Watson (after the founder of IBM), with three industry partners – Apple, Johnson & Johnson and Medtronic – and two smaller start-ups, namely Explorys and Phytel (Lohr, 2015). Explorys is a spin-off from the Cleveland Clinic, and has data on 50 million patients, which can be used to identify patterns in diseases, treatments and outcomes. Phytel makes software to manage patient care and reduce readmission rates to hospitals. IBM plans to use its Watson technology to provide a cloud-based service in order to deliver targeted analyses to hospitals, physicians, insurers, researchers and potentially even individual patients. The ethical and financial implications of this development are staggering, but it also illustrates the gap between industry and academic social science.

The pharmaceutical industry, DTC genetic testing companies such as 23andMe, and technology companies such as IBM and Google, have all seized the potential for enrolling people in their data collection and knowledge production. Sometimes the motives are transparent, to sell drugs or diagnoses. Sometimes the motives are less obvious, as when data are being collected for scientific or market research purposes. Scientific purposes include the aggregation of data for GWAS studies, or the development of new forms of epidemiology, such as with Google Flu Trends.

In 2008, Google started to experiment with using search engine queries to predict disease outbreak. It quickly came to the conclusion that its predictions for influenza outbreaks were as good as, or even better than those made by the US Centers for Disease Control. The report in *Nature* (Butler, 2008) is interesting in terms of method and its combination of different types of data, but it also recognises some of its own limits. For example, Google recognises that it is not only people with influenza symptoms who conduct searches, as sometimes healthy individuals will search on behalf of others, or will react to news stories about flu outbreaks or celebrities coming down with flu. A report in the *New Scientist* in 2014 (Hodson, 2014) suggested that Google Flu Trends had given unreliable results for the preceding three years. It pointed to the lack of transparency in the algorithms used by Google, a common critique of the company, and the fact that it did not disclose the search terms used.

There are other limits. First, we know from research in scientometrics and corpus-based linguistics that words only have meaning in context. Meaning is provided only with hindsight and may not be a good indicator of the future. Words and co-words (relations between words) mean different things depending on context, and meaning may change over time and place. Therefore it is unlikely that search terms by themselves can be used for mapping spatial dynamics of disease outbreak. Second, the temporality of online environments is not easy to determine. Hellsten, Leydesdorff and Wouters (2006) analysed the multiple presents online. They demonstrate that search engines systematically relocate time stamps from the distant past to the present and very recent past, and delete documents from the year to which they were originally assigned. For example, institutional websites that may contain basic information originally uploaded years ago, will be re-stamped with the date of the most recent change. This makes search engines very unreliable historical witnesses, and, relating to the first point, it means there is a loss in the structure of the semantic networks.

We need to remain aware that technology is not a neutral tool that gives researchers unmediated access to data, references, ideas and people. Technology mediates and structures researchers' interactions at all stages of the research process, just as it structures people's efforts to find and share information about their own health. Computational tools, including algorithms, linked data and databases, can be used to harvest data from multiple and diverse sources in order to recombine it for other purposes. While such tools offer many possibilities and may well reduce the time and effort associated with some tasks, they may also render in/visible some literature, information, data, categories, institutions, or people (Bowker and Star, 1999). In this appendix, we have shown how methodological choices bring different kinds of users and non-users into being. We have also seen how digital technologies can affect medical and scholarly research in a variety of ways, all of which may raise ethical and normative questions at any moment in the process and may affect researchers' relationships not only with research participants but also with colleagues, funders and users of research.

References

Asdal, K. and Moser, I. (2012) 'Experiments in context and contexting', *Science, Technology and Human Values*, vol. 37, no. 4, pp. 291–306.

Bakardjieva, M. and Feenberg, A. (2000) 'Involving the virtual subject', *Ethics and Information Technology*, vol. 2, pp. 233–240.

Beaulieu A. (2005) 'Sociable hyperlinks: An ethnographic approach to connectivity', in C. Hine (ed.), *Virtual methods: Issues in social research on the internet*, New York: Berg, pp. 183–197.

Beaulieu, A. and Estalella, A. (2011). 'Rethinking research ethics for mediated settings', *Information, Communication and Society*, vol. 15, no. 1, pp. 23–42.

Berry, D. M. (2004) 'Internet research: Privacy, ethics and alienation: An open source approach', *Internet Research*, vol. 14, no. 4, pp. 323–332.

Bishop, L. (2009) 'Ethical sharing and reuse of qualitative data', *Australian Journal of Social Issues*, vol. 44, no. 3, pp. 255–272.

Bowker, G. C. and Star, S.L. (1999) *Sorting things out: Classification and its consequences*, Cambridge, MA: MIT Press.

Bowker, G. C., Baker, K., Millerand, F. and Ribes, D. (2010) 'Towards information infrastructure studies: Ways of knowing in a networked environment', in J. Hunsinger, L. Klastrup and M. Allen (eds), *International handbook of internet research*, Dordrecht: Springer, pp. 97–118.

boyd, d. and K. Crawford (2012) 'Critical questions for big data: Provocations for a cultural, technological, and scholarly phenomenon', *Information, Communication and Society*, vol. 15, no. 5, pp. 662–679.

Butler, D. (2008) 'Web data predict flu', *Nature*, 19 November, no. 456, pp. 287–288, doi:10.1038/456287a, available at www.nature.com/news/2008/081119/full/

456287a.html (accessed 11 August 2015).

Carusi, A. (2008) 'Data as representation: Beyond anonymity in e-research ethics', *International Journal of Internet Research Ethics*, vol. 1, no. 1, pp. 37–65.

Cherkas, L. F., Harris, J. M., Levinson, E., Spector, T. D. and Prainsack, B. (2010) 'A survey of UK public interest in internet-based personal genome testing', *PLos ONE*, vol. 5, no. 10, article e13473.

Critchley, C., Nicole, D., Otlowski, M. and Chalmers, D. (2015) 'Public reaction to direct-to-consumer online genetic tests. Comparing attitudes, trust and intentions across commercial and conventional providers', *Public Understanding of Science*, vol. 24, no. 6, pp. 731–750.

Denzin, N. and Lincoln, Y. (2011) *The SAGE handbook of qualitative research*, London: Sage.

Do, C. B., Tung, J. Y., Dorfman, E., Kiefer, A. K., Drabant, E. M., Francke, U., Mountain, J. L., Goldman, S. M., Tanner, C. M., Langston, J. W., Wojcicki, A. and Eriksson, N. (2011) 'Web-based genome-wide association study identifies two novel loci and a substantial genetic component for Parkinson's disease', *PLoS Genetics*, vol. 7, no. 6, article e1002141.

Eriksson, N., Macpherson, J. M., Tung, J. Y., Hon, S. L., Naughton, B., Saxonov, S., Avey, L., Wojcicki, A., Pe'er, I. and Mountain, J. (2010) 'Web-based, participant-driven studies yield novel genetic associations for common traits', *PLoS Genetics*, vol. 6, no. 6, pp. 1–20.

Ess, C. (2009) *Digital media ethics*, Cambridge, UK: Polity Press.

Ess, C. and AoIR Ethics Working Committee (2002) *Ethical decision-making and internet research: Recommendations from the AoIR ethics working committee*, Chicago, IL: Association of Internet Researchers, available at http://aoir.org/reports/ethics.pdf.

Genetics and Public Policy Center (2010) *Direct-to-consumer genetic testing companies*, Baltimore, MD: Genetics and Public Policy Center, Johns Hopkins University, www.dnapolicy.org/resources/AlphabetizedDTCGeneticTestingCompanies.pdf (accessed 10 May 2011; archived by WebCite at www.webcitation.org/5znzI162L).

Giddens, A. (1976/1993) *New rules of sociological method*, 2nd edition, Cambridge, UK: Polity Press.

Gubrium, J. F. and Holstein, J. A. (1998) 'Narrative practice and the coherence of personal stories', *The Sociological Quarterly*, vol. 39, no. 1, pp. 163–187.

Hall, S. (ed.) (1997) *Representation: Cultural representation and signifying practices*, London: Sage/Open University.

Harris, R., Wathen, N. and Wyatt, S. (eds) (2010) *Configuring health consumers: Health work and the imperative of personal responsibility*, London: Palgrave Macmillan.

Hellsten, I., Leydesdorff, L. and Wouters, P. (2006) 'Multiple presents: How search engines rewrite the past', *New Media and Society*, vol. 8, no. 6, pp. 901–924.

Hennen, L., Sauter, A. and Van Den Cruyce, E. (2010) 'Direct to consumer genetic testing: Insights from an internet scan', *New Genetics and Society*, vol. 29, no. 2, pp. 167–186.

Henwood, F., Hughes, G., Kennedy, H., Miller, N. and Wyatt, S. (2001) 'Cyborg lives in context. Writing women's technobiographies', in F. Henwood, H. Kennedy and N. Miller (eds), *Cyborg lives? Women's technobiographies*, York: Raw Nerve Press, pp. 11–34.

Hodson, H. (2014) 'Google Flu Trends gets it wrong three years running', *New Scientist*, 13 March, available at www.newscientist.com/article/dn25217-google-flu-trends-gets-it-wrong-three-years-running.html (accessed 16 April 2015).

KNAW (2013) *Responsible research data management and the prevention of scientific misconduct* (also known as the Schuyt report), Amsterdam: Royal Netherlands

Academy of Arts and Sciences (KNAW).

Law, J. (2004) *After method: Mess in social science research*, London: Routledge.

Lee, S. S.-J. and Crawley, L. (2009) 'Research 2.0: Social networking and direct-to-consumer (DTC) genomics', *The American Journal of Bioethics*, vol. 9, pp. 35–44.

Lee, S. S., Vernez, S. L., Ormond, K. E., and Granovetter, M. (2013) 'Attitudes towards Social networking and sharing behaviors among consumers of direct-to-consumer personal genomics', *Journal of Personalized Medicine*, vol. 3, no. 4, pp. 275–287.

Lohr, S. (2015) 'IBM creates Watson Health to analyze medical data', *New York Times*, 13 April, available at http://bits.blogs.nytimes.com/2015/04/13/ibm-creates-watson-health-to-analyze-medical-data/?_r=0 (accessed 15 April 2015).

Lupton D. (1997) 'Foucault and the medicalisation critique', in A. Petersen and R. Bunton (eds), *Foucault, Health and Medicine*, London: Routledge, pp. 94–112.

MacArthur, D., Morley, K. and Jostins, L. (2010) 'Reader survey results: Digging a little deeper', Genomes Unzipped, available at http://genomesunzipped.org/2010/12/reader-survey-results-digging-a-little-deeper.php (accessed 25 August).

McGowan, M. L., Fishman, J. R. and Lambrix, M. A. (2010) 'Personal genomics and individual identities: Motivations and moral imperatives of early users', *New Genetics and Society*, vol. 29, no. 3, pp. 261–290.

Maher, B. (2011) 'Nature readers flirt with personal genomics', *Nature*, vol. 478, p. 19, available at www.nature.com/news/2011/111005/full/478019a.html.

Meyer, E. and Schroeder, R. (2015) *Knowledge machines. Digital transformations of the sciences and humanities*, Cambridge, MA: MIT Press.

Neumann P. J., Cohen, J. T., Hammitt, J. K., Concannon, T. W., Auerbach, H. R. *et al.* (2011) 'Willingness-to-pay for predictive tests with no immediate treatment implications: A survey of US residents', *Health Economics*, vol. 21, no. 3, pp. 238–251.

Nissenbaum, H. (2010) *Privacy in context: Policy and the integrity of social life*, Palo Alto, CA: Stanford University Press.

Oudshoorn, N. and Pinch, T. (eds) (2005) *How users matter: The co-construction of users and technology*, Cambridge, MA: MIT Press.

Prior, L., Evans, M. R. and Prout, H. (2011) 'Talking about colds and flu: The lay diagnosis of two common illnesses among older British people', *Social Science and Medicine*, vol. 73, no. 6, pp. 922–928.

Robison, R. (2009) 'Finding research literature on autism', in K. Börner and M. Stamper (eds), *7th iteration, science maps as visual interfaces to digital libraries*, Bloomington, IN: Places & Spaces: Mapping Science, available at http://scimaps.org/mapdetail/finding_research_lit_126 (accessed 17 April 2015).

Rogers, R. (2013) *Digital methods*, Cambridge, MA: MIT Press.

Ruppert, E., Law, J., and Savage, M. (2013) 'Reassembling social science methods: The challenge of digital devices', *Theory, Culture and Society*, vol. 30, no. 4, pp. 22–46.

Savage, M. and Burrows, R. (2007) 'The coming crisis of empirical sociology', *Sociology*, vol. 41, no. 5, pp. 885–899.

Snee, H., Hine, C., Morey, Y., Roberts, S. and Watson, H. (eds) (2015) *Digital methods for social science: An interdisciplinary guide to research innovation*, Basingstoke: Palgrave Macmillan.

Sterckx, S., Cockbain, J., Howard, H., Huys, I. and Borry, P. (2013) '"Trust is not something you can reclaim easily": Patenting in the field of direct-to-consumer genetic testing', *Genetics in Medicine*, vol. 15, no. 5, pp. 382–387.

Tung, J. Y., Do, C. B., Hinds, D. A., Kiefe, A., Macpherson, J. M., Chowdry, A. B., Francke, U., Naughton, B., Mountain, J., Wojcicki, A. and Eriksson, N. (2011)

'Efficient replication of over 180 genetic associations with self-reported medical data', *PLos ONE*, vol. 6, no. 8, article e23473.

Vernez, S. L., Salari, K., Ormond, K. E. and Lee, S. S. (2013) 'Personal genome testing in medical education: Student experiences with genotyping in the classroom', *Genome Medicine*, vol. 5, no. 3, p. 24.

White, M. (2002) 'Representations or people?', *Ethics and Information Technology*, vol. 4, no. 3, pp. 249–266.

Wouters, P., Beaulieu, A., Scharnhorst, A. and Wyatt, S. (eds) (2013) *Virtual knowledge: Experimenting in the humanities and the social sciences*, Cambridge, MA: MIT Press.

Wyatt, S. (2012) 'Ethics of e-research in social sciences and humanities', in D. Heider and A. Massanari (eds), *Digital ethics, research and practice*, New York: Peter Lang, pp. 5–20.

Wyatt, S., Harris, A. and Kelly, S. (2016) 'Controversy goes online: Schizophrenia genetics on Wikipedia', *Science and Technology Studies*, vol. 29, no. 1, pp. 13–29.

Appendix B

Direct-to-consumer genetic testing websites

In December 2010, a list of websites for companies offering genetic testing services to consumers was compiled by Anna Harris after consulting recently published literature (e.g. Hennen *et al.*, 2010, and a list of companies compiled by the Genetics and Public Policy Center (2010). This was supplemented with online searches using various search engines (Google, Yahoo, Bing and Ask) by entering terms such as 'genetic testing' and 'direct to consumer genetic test'; and TouchGraph, a web link visualisation tool, by typing in the term 'genetic testing'. This generated a total of 52 websites.

Direct-to-consumer psychiatric-only genetic testing sites

NeuroMark
Psynomics
Suregene

General direct-to-consumer genetic testing sites with tests related to psychiatric conditions

23andMe
Navigenics
DeCODEme
Knome
Genelex
Pathway Genomics
Counsyl
GeneDX
Genova Diagnostics
Suracell
Consumer Genetics
Graceful Earth
Kimball Genetics
Mygenome
Gene Planet

EasyDNA
My Gene Profile
Health Genetics Centre

Direct-to-consumer genetic testing sites not offering tests for psychiatric conditions

Genomic Health
Myriad
Carolyn Katzin's DNA diet
DNAPrint Genomics
Cygene direct
Eastern Biotech and Lifesciences
GATC
Genetic Health
HairDx
HealthCheckUSA
HIVGene
Know your genetics
Inherent Health (Interleukin Genetics)
MDL Labs
Medichecks
Atlas genes
BioMarker Pharmaceuticals
DNACardioCheck
DNA Dimensions
DNA Plus
Enterolab
Nimble Diagnostics

Genetic testing websites where it is not clear if it is direct-to-consumer or which diseases they test for

Burc Genetic Diagnostic Centre
Genelink
Salugen
Health Tests Direct
SeqWright
DNA Traits
Genomic Express
Inneova
The Genetic Testing Laboratories

Reference

Hennen, L., Sauter, A. and Van Den Cruyce, E. (2010) 'Direct to consumer genetic testing: Insights from an internet scan', *New Genetics and Society*, vol. 29, no. 2, pp. 167–186.

Index